100 Questions & Answers About Depression

Ava T. Albrecht, MD
New York University School of Medicine

Charles Herrick, MD
New York Medical College

JONES AND BARTLETT PUBLISHERS
Sudbury, Massachusetts
BOSTON TORONTO LONDON SINGAPORE

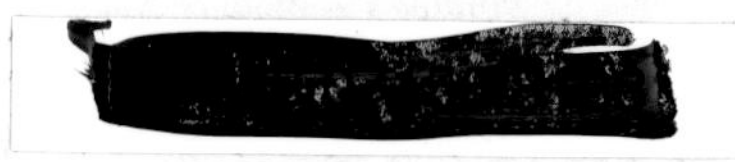

World Headquarters
Jones and Bartlett Publishers
40 Tall Pine Drive
Sudbury, MA 01776
info@jbpub.com
www.jbpub.com

Jones and Bartlett Publishers Canada
2406 Nikanna Road
Mississauga, ON L5C 2W6
CANADA

Jones and Bartlett Publishers International
Barb House, Barb Mews
London W6 7PA
UK

Jones and Bartlett's books and products are available through most bookstores and online booksellers. To contact Jones and Bartlett Publishers directly, call 800-832-0034, fax 978-443-8000, or visit our website www.jbpub.com.

Substantial discounts on bulk quantities of Jones and Bartlett's publications are available to corporations, professional associations, and other qualified organizations. For details and specific discount information, contact the special sales department at Jones and Bartlett via the above contact information or send an email to specialsales@jbpub.com.

Library of Congress Cataloging-in-Publication Data
Albrecht, Ava T.
100 questions and answers about depression / Ava T. Albrecht, Charles Herrick.
p. cm.
Includes bibliographical references and index.
ISBN-13: 978-0-7637-4567-7
1. Depression, Mental—Popular works. I. Title: One hundred questions and answers about depression. II. Herrick, Charles. III. Title.
RC537.A42 2006
616.85'27—dc22

2005006477

The authors, editor, and publisher have made every effort to provide accurate information. However, they are not responsible for errors, omissions, or for any outcomes related to the use of the contents of this book and take no responsibility for the use of the products described. Treatments and side effects described in this book may not be applicable to all patients; likewise, some patients may require a dose or experience a side effect that is not described herein. The reader should confer with his or her own physician regarding specific treatments and side effects. Drugs and medical devices are discussed that may have limited availability controlled by the Food and Drug Administration (FDA) for use only in a research study or clinical trial. The drug information presented has been derived from reference sources, recently published data, and pharmaceutical research data. Research, clinical practice, and government regulations often change the accepted standard in this field. When consideration is being given to use of any drug in the clinical setting, the health care provider or reader is responsible for determining FDA status of the drug, reading the package insert, reviewing prescribing information for the most up-to-date recommendations on dose, precautions, and contraindications, and determining the appropriate usage for the product. This is especially important in the case of drugs that are new or seldom used.

Production Credits
Executive Publisher: Chris Davis
Production Director: Amy Rose
Editorial Assistant: Kathy Richardson
Production Assistant: Alison Meier
Marketing Associate: Laura Kavigian
Manufacturing Buyer: Therese Bräuer
Composition: Northeast Compositors
Cover Design: Colleen Halloran
Printing and Binding: Malloy, Inc.
Cover Printing: Malloy, Inc.

Printed in the United States of America
09 08 07 06 05 10 9 8 7 6 5 4 3 2 1

We dedicate this book to our spouses,
Joseph and Ana Cristina,
for their steadfast support and contribution.

We give special thanks to
Anne Smith and Anthony Sansone,
for their observations and personal accounts
of living with depression.

Contents

Foreword

The attempt to communicate difficult psychiatric material to the general public is often characterized by oversimplification. Frequently, it turns into a kind of pop psychology, which belongs in the advice to the love-lorn column of your daily newspaper. At other times, the communication becomes so complex that it becomes incomprehensible. It is indeed difficult to take medical material and render it into a form that does honor to the integrity of the material and shows respect for the intelligence of the audience. The authors of this volume have been remarkably effective in achieving their goals.

The approach in this book is unusual. The authors have taken a series of questions that are likely to be asked by a lay person seeking an understanding of how the mind works and how it goes awry. The questions range from "what are emotions" to "why was I given a particular drug?" There is also logic to the sequence of questions as they progress in complexity and become more clinical in nature. The authors maintain a strikingly consistent tone throughout the volume. One could disagree with the content in specific areas, but at no time does it verge into bias. There is a consistent perspective that recognizes both the biology and the psychology of the individual. The authors are nonideologic. They recognize the inherent complexity of the human being and that the different ways of conceptualizing that complexity refer to disciplines and not to truth. It has been said that God did not create the world along the lines of a university's department structure. This is particularly true when one looks at the distinction between mind and body, which although useful should not be reified.

Again, the format of this volume is unusual, as it is not divided into chapters and topics but rather into a series of questions. Some readers may be more interested in one question than another, but I believe that most people would benefit from a careful reading of this small volume. In my opinion, it is extraordinarily balanced and not polemical, and I highly recommend this book for anyone interested in learning more about depression.

Robert Cancro, M.D., Med.D.Sc.
Lucius N. Littauer Professor of Psychiatry and Chairman
New York University School of Medicine

Introduction

100 Questions & Answers is a series of books that addresses patient and family concerns on a variety of health related topics. To date however, the majority of books in this series have been on various cancer diagnoses and other physical illnesses. Depression, however, is found in nearly a quarter of persons receiving care in a primary care setting. To that end, it only seemed sensible to develop a similar book on the topic of depression. Writing such a book in this format has been both challenging and rewarding. Many concepts need to be included that are rather abstract and do not always fit neatly within a structure so well suited to physical illnesses with well defined physical descriptors and anatomy. We believe, however, that we have accomplished the task of communicating difficult-to-understand material on a complex subject that still remains in many ways a mystery. Not so long ago, many individuals suffered from depression and mental illness in general, quietly and discreetly. With the introduction of Prozac in the late 1980s, the treatment of depression became a real and tangible option for many people. But ironically, as antidepressants are becoming one of the most prescribed medications in history, depression remains one of the most misunderstood illnesses of our time. Fear is often behind the misunderstanding. The fear often revolves around an admission of losing one's mind when being diagnosed with depression or of losing one's mind from the prescribed psychotropic medication. Such fears persist because of continued confusion regarding the boundaries between the body and the soul. Fundamental assumptions about what is and is not disease versus personal responsibility are called into question, as are the interaction between mind and

brain, the differences between universal human feelings and pathology, and the conceptions of ourselves as being in control over our emotions and behavior. For many people depression continues to be a source of shame as it suggests a weakness of the will. All these reasons create obstacles for people seeking psychiatric attention and asking questions that may reflect negatively on them. The negative stigma of mental illness, no matter how much modern science has attempted to eradicate it, remains strong in our popular culture. In writing this book, we have attempted to answer basic questions readers might have after being diagnosed with depression, or that families might have regarding their loved one. In starting with basic information about the brain, we hope to place into perspective the role the brain plays in the development of depression, and thus its biological underpinnings. In doing so, it is our hope that readers of our book will feel less ashamed and more empowered to attend to their illness, as they would any other medical diagnosis. This is not to undermine, however, the importance of real-life circumstances in the development of depression, as genes do not work in a vacuum. As the environment can influence the likelihood of developing cancer, hypertension, or heart disease, so too the environment influences the development of mental illness, even in the presence of strong genetic influences. A person with heart disease in the family can reduce personal risk by modifying the influence of external stressors on the heart (e.g. quitting smoking, following a low-fat diet). Similarly, a person with depression in the family can reduce personal risk by modifying the influence of stress on the brain (e.g. attending therapy, getting exercise).

We hope to provide the reader with clear, matter-of-fact answers to a multitude of questions that one might have but has been afraid to ask. Some questions have straightforward, simple answers. Others do not. Differences of opinion among clinicians in regards to some of the answers may exist, but we have attempted to present the various aspects that can be considered in any question, so that ultimately the reader can be fully informed when seeking and/or continuing his or her own treatment. There are bound to be questions the reader will have that may not have been fully answered in our book. In today's society, there are vast resources available to laypersons to become involved in their own medical care. Take advantage of these resources. Ask your doctor questions. Get the help that you need.

Ava T. Albrecht, MD
Charles Herrick, MD

Biography

Three years after Anne Smith was married, her husband suffered a major depressive episode. At the time, she had a 1-year-old child and was expecting another. Her husband recovered and resumed his career and family life, but he has had to remain on medication and continues to be monitored by a psychiatrist, attending therapy sessions regularly.

When Anne's daughter was 13 years old, she suffered a traumatic medical event and, in the aftermath, became depressed. Her depression worsened throughout adolescence, and despite medical intervention, she experienced her first episode of mania when she was 18 years old. She spent 3 months in a psychiatric hospital. Once she was released, it took 2 years of intensive treatment before she could consider resuming her academic career.

She continues to struggle with the illness, and Anne is in close communication with the doctors who are overseeing her treatment away from home. Although her independence has been compromised to the degree of extra support she requires, she has gained so much by returning to the life of a college student and testing her limits instead of allowing the illness to limit her.

At the age of 9 years, one of Anne's sons began to show signs of depression. He was treated for depression with medication and responded rapidly to treatment. Within a year he was off medication and back to normal. At the age of 15, he again began to exhibit symptoms of depression. After months of therapy, his conditioned worsened, and a psychiatric evaluation indicated bipolar disorder. Given his sister's history with the illness, the doctor treated him aggressively, and he responded well to medication while continuing therapy sessions.

All three members of Anne's family will remain on medications indefinitely. The family is grateful for the care that each doctor has provided and the dedication each has shown. They are thankful to be living in an era when medication to treat these conditions is available.

Anne's family experience with this illness has been a painful and often terrifying journey, affecting several generations. There has been an ebb and flow to the illness, even with medication. What the medication has allowed is the dynamic of the disease to fall within a livable radius. Despite a family history of depression and suicide, Anne is hopeful that with vigilance, astute medical intervention, and the unwavering love and support of family and friends, the outcome for those in her family who suffer from depression will be to experience what it is to be fully engaged in life.

Anthony Sansone was born in the late 1940s into a large extended family who resided in the same town. An unusually avid reader in his family, he was often scoffed at by family members as a child, but opted still to pursue his educational goals. He obtained a B.S. in history and foreign languages followed by a Master's degree in education/history, and had further advanced study in foreign languages. Anthony is multilingual and currently works as a teacher of foreign language. He enjoys walking and exercising and loves reading. He began receiving mental health services in 1974 while working as a teacher; he has been in therapy and has received medication for depression and anxiety. In 1993, he was diagnosed and treated for testicular cancer, which exacerbated his depression and anxiety. He still recalls his experience with cancer as a significant emotional trauma in his life. A survivors group was extremely helpful in dealing with the illness and his reaction to it, feeling highly devastated by the diagnosis. Presently, under the care of his psychiatrist, symptoms of depression and anxiety are under reasonable control as Anthony continues to work and enjoy life.

PART ONE

The Basics

What are emotions, and why do we have them?

What is the difference between thoughts and feelings?

How does the brain affect behavior and regulate emotional states?

More . . .

1. What are emotions, and why do we have them?

No absolutely agreed on definition for emotions exists. Many dictionaries refer to "feelings" or "moods" when defining the word; this further begs the question of what they are. Scientists who attempt to study emotional phenomena characterize them in terms of their particular interest, and thus, definitions change depending on whether the scientist is studying the biological, psychological, or social basis of emotions. This, of course, further complicates the understanding of emotions.

Historically, the mind was thought to be separate from the body and part of the soul. In fact, *psyche* is the Greek root for "soul." With the advent of a more scientific understanding of the brain and mind, some scientists attempt to liken the mind to software and the brain to hardware. In actuality, however, it is not quite so simple. A simultaneous change in brain activity accompanies every change in thought, feeling, perception, or action. Today, scientists increasingly appreciate the fact that no sharp demarcation exists between the brain and the mind.

Despite the fact that mind and brain are essentially unified, drawing a boundary between the two allows for practical differences between them to be conceptualized in everyday lives. For example, such a boundary permits distinction between acts and motives. Distinguishing acts from motives helps with negotiation through everyday social interactions. For example, consider the feelings generated when standing in line and having your toes stepped on. With the immediate sensation of pain comes the feelings of shock, surprise, and probably anger. The feelings experienced are immediately followed by an assessment of the person's motives or state of mind. Action on that assessment is guided by feelings. Emotions therefore serve to engage the body to act in some manner. The manner on which an action is taken usually carries some survival value to a given individual.

Thus, lack of emotions could be likened to the lack of physical pain sensation. There would be numbness to the environment and thus problems in interacting with it appropriately. Without the ability to feel anger, joy, sorrow, fear, or love, humans would be incapable of generating priorities to action. Emotions help to prioritize—to decide when to act and when not to act. Without such abilities, choosing between arrays of decisions that are confronted on a daily basis would be unfeasible.

2. What is the difference between thoughts and feelings?

Emotions or feelings are often distinguished from thoughts. Emotions are typically considered the irrational or animal part of humans, whereas thoughts are the rational. Strong feelings such as anger, joy, fear, and sadness result in behaviors that do not seem to always serve one's interests. Thoughts are the words in the head that give mental content to hopes, dreams, and desires and allow for reasoning and weighing of options so that an assessment of consequences can be made before actions are taken.

Scientists now know through the use of experiments and clinical observation that thoughts, feelings, and perceptions coexist as a unified whole and cannot be easily teased apart. Thus, every thought is given a positive or negative emotional valence that allows us to prioritize our actions on those thoughts. Evidence in support of that comes from the fields of neurology and the computer sciences. **Neurologic** studies show that people who suffered brain damage that cuts thoughts off from feelings are unable to prioritize a list of preferences and act on them in order to achieve even the simplest of goals. Even simple tasks, such as choosing a restaurant, become impossible because of entrapment in a never-ending cost–benefit analysis of numerous and conflicting options. Similarly, computer programmers have struggled to develop simple **algorithms** that can generate decisions, appropriately weighing all of the costs and benefits without becoming literally buried underneath an infinite loop of ones and zeros. Emotions are therefore a necessary piece that works with thoughts in decision making and hence planning of future goals.

Neurological

referring to all matters of the nervous system that includes brain, brainstem, spinal cord, and peripheral nerves.

Algorithm

a sequence of steps to follow when approaching a particular problem.

3. How does the brain affect behavior and regulate emotional states?

Emotions are regulated by the complex interaction between various brain components and the environment in a feedback loop that allows for both the environment to impact brain structure and function and the brain to impact on the environment through action. More than being a two-way street, however, the brain is more like a superhighway. This highway consists of a variety of environmental inputs (some that are available to our consciousness but many that are not) and our ultimate responses to those inputs. Environmental inputs available to our consciousness are those that we typically associate with the five senses: sight, smell, taste, hearing, and touch. The mere words conjure up a myriad of **emotional memories** for experiences that we have had in the past. A certain odor or song can suddenly take a person back to a previous relationship or situation. The connection between a current environmental cue and memories is caused by actual structural changes in the brain. In fact, long-term memories are long term because of those structural changes. The brain is not a computer but is a dynamic organ that is capable of physical change throughout one's life.

Emotional memory
a memory evoked by a sensory experience.

Although sensory inputs are generally obvious, a multitude of environmental inputs occurs without conscious awareness. The brain is also constantly monitoring our body's internal environment, the available nutrients and chemicals, blood pressure, pulse, temperature, and respiration, and it adjusts itself accordingly. It is also monitoring the external environment in ways that are not immediately apparent. These unconscious inputs can affect the emotional state in ways that are not always obvious.

Interpretations of these inputs that prompt actions are also influenced by two important factors influencing the brain long before inputs are received. Built into the brain are sets of biases, some of which are determined by **genes** and the biological (uterine) environment in which development occurs and others by past experiences. Although genes do not cause behavior, they are the foundation for a person's entire organic make-up. Genes code for proteins, which are the building blocks for both the structure and function of the human organism. Genes guide **neuroanatomy**, and in turn,

Gene
DNA sequence that codes for a specific protein or that regulates other genes. Genes are heritable.

Neuroanatomy
the structural makeup of the nervous system and nervous tissue.

Neurophysiology
the part of science devoted specifically to the physiology, or function and activities, of the nervous system.

Neuronal plasticity
the act of nerve growth and change as a result of learning.

Depression
a medical condition associated with changes in thoughts, moods, and behaviors.

Constitution
referring to a person's biopsychological make-up, that is, the personality and the traits.

Brainstem
the anatomical part of the brain that contains the major centers that regulate sleep, appetite, blood pressure, temperature, and respiration.

Basal ganglia
a region of the brain consisting of three groups of nerve cells collectively responsible for control of movement.

neuroanatomy and **neurophysiology** guide actions. Past experiences, on the other hand, are literally carved into brains through a process conceptualized as **neuronal plasticity**. Nerves are literally pruned away like tree branches through learning and experience as the brain attempts to create more efficient and faster communication pathways through those repeated experiences. By the nature of genetics and developmental experiences, people are biased to respond to the environment in certain ways. Although bias can predispose people toward negative actions and may be one of the mechanisms behind the development of some types of **depression**, it is merely biology's way of simplifying behavioral strategies to create more rapid and efficient actions. Without emotions, one cannot prioritize; priorities to action must be linked to a preconceived template of what one considers important in decision making. This is the bias based on one's emotional experiences and **constitutional** nature (genes and non-genetic biological effects).

In terms of defining the specific areas of the brain—or the anatomical locations—that control emotions, the division of regions is not clear cut. One of the oldest and easiest to understand (but not necessarily the most accurate) theories divides the brain into three regions or layers. The most primitive is the **brainstem** and **basal ganglia**, followed by the **limbic system** and then the rational brain that is comprised of the cortex. The first layer is that part responsible for self-preservation. It is where the "**fight or flight**" response is generated in response to perceived danger. The brainstem is also where control of certain **visceral** or "vegetative" functions (sleep, appetite, libido, heart rate, blood pressure, etc.), are generated. The limbic region (from the Latin word *limbus* for, ring, or surrounding, as it forms a kind of border around the brainstem) is better known as the reward center, where emotions or feelings such as anger, fear, love, hate, joy, and sadness originate. The limbic system is also responsible for some aspects of personal identity as related to the emotional power of memory. The third cerebral region is considered the "rational brain," which is capable of producing symbolic language and developing intellectual tasks such as reading, writing, and performing mathematical calculations. These neuroanatomic distinctions are really not that distinct but are integrated into function as a unified whole such that an assumption cannot be made of any one system taking priority over the other. The notions of brain regions as "primitive versus advanced" and "inferior versus superior" have not been supported by modern science. Brain structures are not hierarchical but are egalitarian. Brain function is more akin to an orchestra rather than the more common notion of a military command center, as each component is required for the entire symphony to work where the conductor is merely a "ghost in the machine."

Limbic system
the part of the brain thought to be related to feeding, mating, and most importantly to emotion and memory of emotional events.

Fight or flight
a reaction in the body that occurs in response to an immediate threat.

Visceral
a bodily sensation usually referencing the gut; also a feeling or thought attributed to intuition rather than reason, such as "a gut instinct."

4. What is mental illness? What is a major mental illness?

Before **mental illness** can be defined, the concept of illness needs to be understood more completely. As medicine has become increasingly driven by technologic advances, the concept of disease has supplanted the concept of illness. Medicine is driven by a need for

Mental illness
a medical condition defined by functional symptoms that impairs social, academic, and occupational function, with as yet no specific pathophysiology.

objective evidence and removal of subjective experience. Subjective data, although they can help inform our understanding of diseases, are by their very nature experienced only by the one subject, rather than witnessed by a community, and thus, they are inherently unreliable. In contrast, major advances have come from objective, experimental approaches to various diseases and their treatments. With the cost of healthcare skyrocketing, making healthcare dollars less and less available to treat any given disease, simple economic necessity dictates that we spend money on things that yield results. With a finite number of dollars, money is therefore spent on diseases that can be defined and cured.

Humans, however, are more than just their diseases. To be human is to experience the disease in a unique way that other humans cannot experience. To be human with a disease is to suffer from an illness. Having an illness is a subjective experience that may be easily dismissed as less important than the objective facts of the disease. In treating individual patients, doctors address both disease and illness; one piece of that treatment is the elimination or control of the disease. Healing, on the other hand, requires more than just the elimination of disease; it requires an understanding of the person's experience with the disease in the form of their illness and the elimination of that as well.

Mental illness can be complicated to define, as it is generally based on the subjective experience of those suffering from it. Fortunately, the field of psychiatry has experienced technologic advances, and the numbers of effective psychiatric therapies available to treat mental illness have exploded in the past 10 years. Unfortunately, although the scientific theories have continued to advance our understanding of possible underlying causes, little to no clinically useful objective evidence remains to validate the disease concept. This is why mental illness is so devastating to individuals suffering from it and remains so stigmatized by those who little understand it. Consider the different feelings experienced by a patient who sees his or her internist for a variety of physical complaints for which all of the testing is negative and he or she is left languishing in the helpless idea that his or her complaints are "all in his or her head," whereas a patient visiting the psychiatrist with the same array of complaints is provided with a medical explanation of his or her illness and feels reassured that it is "not all in his or her head." Webster's dictionary defines mental illness as a "disease of the mind," illustrating the struggle to identify boundaries between disease versus illness and mind versus body. Such a distinction has its utility but leads to the shame and stigmatization that exists for those suffering from mental illness.

Mental illness is better thought of in the less pejorative sense of being a disease, if merely for the fact that it brings aid and comfort to those who suffer from it. Certainly enough biological evidence exists to argue strongly for this definition even if no clinical testing exists. What defines the "menu" of symptoms listed in the *Diagnostic and Statistical Manual of Mental Disorders, Fourth Edition, Text-Revised* (DSM-IV-TR) is not just having the list of symptoms outlined in each disorder, but rather showing the impact that those symptoms have on one's life in terms of distress and disability. It is that universal inclusion criteria (along with the universal exclusion criteria of "not due to a medical condition or toxic reaction") that define the boundaries between normal variant, mentally ill, and physically ill. Defining the differences between the normal and pathologic serves to avoid the subjectivity that can occur when defining illness of thought, emotions, or behavior. Any condition defined in the DSM-IV-TR is considered a mental illness or disorder.

Many terms are thrown about today in popular culture that are used to distinguish between types of mental illnesses, most of which stem from the previous discussion regarding the stigmatization and shame that accompany the diagnosis. Such terms include, but are not limited to, behavior disorder, brain disorder, minimal brain dysfunction, nervous breakdown, neurosis, psychosis, panic disorder, depression, schizophrenia, **personality disorder**, character disorder, major mental illness, minor mental illness, and "biologically based condition." Most of these terms have more than one meaning depending on who defines them. These terms may be defined by the following:

Personality disorder

maladaptive behavior patterns that persist throughout the life span, which cause functional impairments.

- Media and popular culture
- Politics that ultimately influence an insurance company's financial responsibility to pay for the treatment
- The legal system to aid the criminal courts' decision to find someone not guilty by reason of insanity
- The psychiatric and psychological communities

First, in popular culture and media, mental illness is defined by the idea that one is either "crazy" or not. Terms such as "insane," "deranged," "demented," "mentally ill," "psychotic," and "schizophrenic" are most often associated with some appalling violent or criminal act that seems to lack any understandable motive that can be discovered by either the police or the press. In this situation, "crazy" substitutes for the lack of apparent motive. No matter how many times the argument is made that the mentally ill are no more violent than society at large, the press never stops from pointing out when someone is mentally ill after being arrested for a heinous criminal act. Some of these terms, such as schizophrenia, do have specific psychiatric definitions that are part of the DSM-IV-TR. Some include legal terms (such as insanity) that only the courts can determine. The media and popular culture, however, define all in pejorative terms that carry clear moral connotations. It is such definitions that lead patients to avoid a psychiatrist's office for fear of being labeled crazy or mentally ill.

Second, political, legal, or economic definitions of mental illness are meant to protect people from arbitrary actions by virtue of their illness. This is where the terms biologically based, behavior disorder, and insanity derive. Because of the broad reach of behavior making up the definitions of mental illness where no validated biological tests exist, the potential for abuse in our social system is rife. As a result, legal and political definitions were instituted to protect individuals and organizations from that potential abuse. To protect individuals, the definition of biologically based was established in order to force insurers to pay for their treatment. These include such DSM-IV-TR disorders as schizophrenia, major depressive disorder, and **bipolar disorder**. Alternatively, behavior disorders are

Bipolar disorder
a mental illness defined by episodes of mania or hypomania, classically alternating with episodes of depression.

not considered biologically based from the insurers' perspective and thus are the responsibility of the individual and are not subject to third-party payment. Insanity is a strictly legal definition that only the courts can determine. It may be informed by the fact that an individual is suffering from a mental illness, but that is only part of the equation. One may suffer from schizophrenia but rob a grocery store for purely financial reasons. He or she is not judged insane; although from the point of view of psychiatry, he or she has a mental illness, and from the point of view of the popular press, that person can be called "crazy."

Definitions that interest scientists and clinicians the most are of the third type, specific operational criteria attempting to codify mental and behavioral phenomena in a pattern that has a specific etiology (cause), diagnostic symptom list (pattern), and prognosis (result). The history of attempting to classify and understand mental illness is as long as the history of medicine itself. Distinctions between biologically based, psychologically based, and socially based are relevant only in so far as attempts are made to understand each individual, biological, psychological, and social element that goes into causing each disorder. This does not mean that psychiatry is without its own arbitrary distinctions. A distinction can be made between major mental illnesses and personality disorders, classified as Axis I and Axis II diagnoses in the DSM-IV-TR. The two axes distinguish between major mental illnesses or states that can wax and wane with time and treatment and personality disorders, or traits, that are generally considered to be enduring and unresponsive to biological therapies. States change. Traits endure. This distinction is one of the "useful fictions" that inform our understanding of behavior in general and mental illness more specifically. The line between state and trait is very gray but has allowed psychiatry to focus historically and to set limits on what can be accurately defined and treated. In the past, personality disorders were considered not changeable and not treatable. As science has advanced, however, there has been a discovery that certain elements of personality do change with time and are improved with treatment. Insurers and the courts, however, continue to make such distinctions, as this is what is generally meant by the difference between biologically based versus behavior disorder or mentally ill versus personality disordered.

5. What is the DSM-IV-TR?

The DSM-IV-TR (*Diagnostic and Statistical Manual of Mental Disorders, Fourth Edition, Text-Revised*) is considered the standard diagnostic manual for establishing the diagnosis of various mental disorders. Of note, in its introduction, a few caveats are outlined. First, mental disorder implies a distinction from physical disorders that is a relic of mind/body dualism. Second, "'mental disorder' lacks a consistent operational definition that covers all situations." Third, the categorical approach has limitations in that discrete entities are assumed when in fact there are no absolute boundaries dividing one disorder from another. Fourth, the criteria for each disorder serve as guidelines only and should not be applied in either a "cookbook fashion" or in an "excessively flexible" manner. Finally, the purpose of the manual is primarily to enhance agreement among clinicians and investigators and is not to imply that any "condition meets legal or other non-medical criteria for what constitutes mental disease, mental disorder, or mental disability" (see Introduction and Cautionary Statement of DSM-IV-TR).

It is critical to keep these caveats in mind, as it is easy to get caught in a physician's diagnosis, believing that it is set in stone, which it is not. As new information is acquired in treatment, the diagnosis and **treatment plan** may change. Additionally, it is not uncommon for clinicians to disagree on the diagnosis because of the previously mentioned caveats. When reading the various criteria individually, it is easy to identify with many of them and jump to the conclusion that one has the described condition. Only time and the guidance of a skilled clinician who is probing and comprehensive in his or her questioning will help to establish a diagnosis that leads to an effective treatment plan. The ability to establish a diagnosis is important in developing a treatment plan that restores one's health, and if the treatment plan fails, the first order of business is to reconsider the diagnosis.

6. *How do chemicals work in the brain?*

The brain is a complex organ that is comprised of **gray matter** and **white matter**. Gray matter consists of the cell bodies of **neurons** and other support cells, and the white matter consists of long tracts of **axons** that run between the neurons. Figure 1 shows an illustration of a neuron. Different areas of the brain have somewhat specific functions. For example, the **motor cortex** controls voluntary movements of the body, and the sensory cortex processes information to the senses. Different areas of the brain communicate with other areas nearby as well as more distantly. Information

Treatment plan
the plan agreed on by patient and clinician that will be implemented to treat a mental illness.

Gray matter
the part of the brain that contains the nerve cell bodies, such as the cerebral cortex.

White matter
tracts in the brain that consist of sheaths (called myelin) covering long nerve fibers.

Neuron
a nerve cell made up of a cell body with extensions called the dendrites and the axon.

Axon
a single fiber of a nerve cell through which a message is sent via an electrical impulse to a receiving neuron.

Motor cortex
portion of the cerebral cortex that is directly related to voluntary movement.

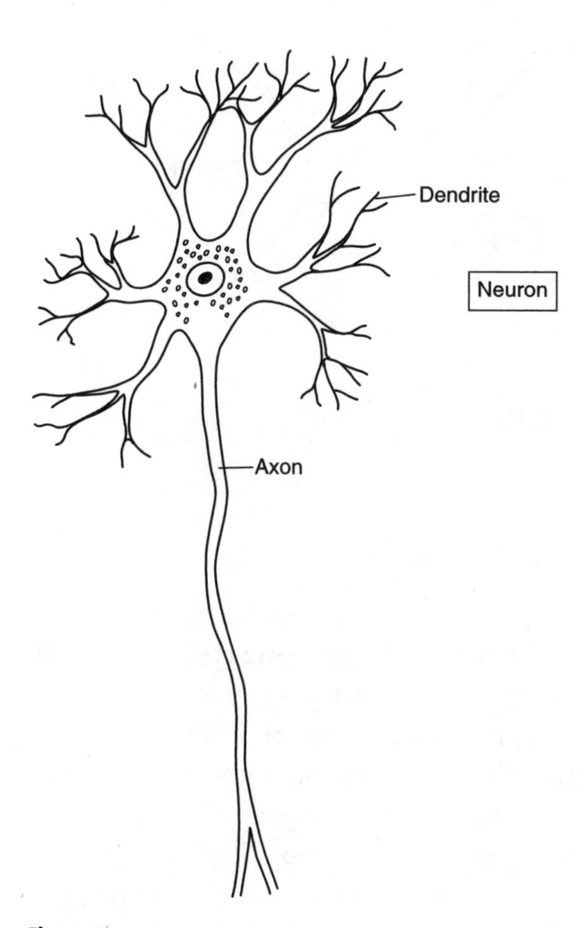

Figure 1

travels via the axons of the neurons within the white matter areas of the brain.

The brain contains billions of neurons, which interact with each other **electrochemically**. This means that when a nerve is stimulated, a series of chemical events occur that in turn create an electrical impulse. The resulting impulse propagates down the nerve length known as the axon and causes a release of chemicals called **neurotransmitters** into a space between the

Electrochemically
the mechanism by which signals are transmitted neurologically.

Neurotransmitter
chemical in the brain that is released by nerve cells to send a message to other cells via the cell receptors.

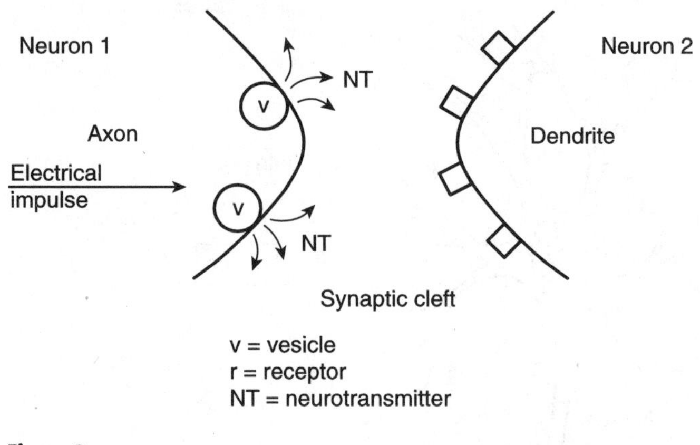

Figure 2

stimulated nerve and the nerve that it wishes to communicate with, known as the **synaptic cleft** (Figure 2). The neurotransmitters interact with **receptors** on the second nerve, either stimulating or inhibiting them. The interaction between the neurotransmitters and receptors can be likened to a key interacting with a lock where the neurotransmitter or "key" engages the receptor or "lock," causing it to "open." This opening is really a series of chemical changes within the second nerve that either causes that nerve to "fire" or "not fire." Thus, brain activity is the result of an orchestrated series of nerves firing or not firing in a binary fashion. In that sense, it is much like a computer where very complicated processes begin their lives as a series of 1s or 0s (on or off, fire or do not fire).

Synaptic cleft
the junction between two neurons where neurotransmitters are released.

Receptor
a protein on a cell on which chemicals bind to cause an electrochemical message for a certain action to be taken by that cell.

After the nerve fires, thereby releasing neurotransmitters into the synaptic cleft, the neurotransmitters must be removed from the area in order to turn the signal off. There are two ways that these chemicals can be removed in order to turn the signal off. The first is by destroying the chemical through the use of another chemical known as an **enzyme** with that specific purpose in mind. The second is by pumping the chemical back into the nerve that released it by using another special chemical known as a transporter or transport pump. The process of pumping chemicals back into the nerve is known as reuptake (Figure 2). It is important to understand these basic principals of neurophysiology because *all* psychoactive compounds, whether neurotransmitters, hormones, medications, or addictive drugs, involve one or more of these simple mechanisms.

Enzyme
a protein made in the body that serves to break down or create other molecules.

7. *What is depression?*

Depression is a medical condition that affects a person's thoughts and feelings as well as the body. It can be associated with various physical problems, such as sleep, appetite, energy, libido, and a variety of bodily discomforts. Research increasingly argues for the fact that depression is not a condition resulting from personal or moral weakness but is a treatable illness. Although it is often associated with feelings of sadness or the "blues," it is not the same thing. The best way to characterize clinical depression from normal sadness is to think of the term depression in a global, bodily sense, where there is a reduction in **physiological** activity across a variety of physical systems, including emotion and cognition. Although **stressors** can trigger an episode of depression, the stressful life event alone does not cause the condition. Anyone is susceptible to depression, although certain populations are at a higher risk. Untreated, depression can last for weeks, months, or years. Many people have recurrent episodes. As with

Physiological
pertaining to functions and activities of the living matter, such as organs, tissues, or cells.

Stressors
environmental influences on the body and mind that can have gradual adverse effects.

any illness, both **morbidity** and **mortality** are associated with depression. Morbidity is a result of the functional impairment that a person experiences in areas of work, school, and relationships. Mortality is due to death by suicide or accidental death because of the functional impairments (e.g., car accident, illicit drug use, poor nutrition, and neglect of health).

Morbidity

the impact a particular disease process or illness has on one's social, academic, or occupational functioning.

Mortality

death secondary to illness or disease.

The majority of people who are depressed will respond to treatment, and thus, it is unwarranted for anyone to suffer through an episode. The affected person may believe that no one else suffers in the same way and that he or she is alone in having depression. However, depression is a common illness around the world. The lifetime **prevalence** for depression is approximately 15%, and in any given 1-year period, there are 18.8 million adults in the United States who suffer from depression. Close to 25% of persons seeking medical treatment in their primary care doctor's office suffer from depression. Not only does depression have a personal cost on individuals and their families, it has a significant cost on society. As many people who are depressed do not seek treatment, the cost of untreated depression to society runs into tens of billions of dollars, in part because of decreased productivity at work and overuse of primary healthcare services. Only approximately half of people with major depression ever receive specific treatment, as symptoms of depression may be inappropriately dismissed as understandable reactions to stress, evidence of personal weakness, or an attempt to receive secondary gain (such as attention from others or disability payments).

Prevalence

ratio of the frequency of cases in the population in a given time period of a particular event to the number of persons in the population at risk for the event.

8. What causes depression?

Anthony's comment:

While depression is not 100% heritable, I think it often runs in families even if one is not aware of it being present in other family members. In the early 1970s, due to severe anxiety over my identity, I went to see a psychiatrist, and received treatment with medication. I needed something that allowed me to function. I was the only one in my extended family however who ever sought professional help to deal with anxiety and depression. As a result, I was labeled with everything under the sun. But, while no one else has actually been diagnosed with depression in my family, it is my impression that there are in fact family members who deal with depression and anxiety, but due to unawareness, stigma, etc. have not been formally diagnosed or treated.

The causes of depression are not easily defined. When speaking of cause, it is typical to think in terms of infections of the lungs causing pneumonia or of cigarette smoking causing lung cancer. In actuality, most medical conditions cannot be so easily defined as having clearly linked causes. In fact, it took many years of statistical analysis before scientists could demonstrate a clear causal link between cigarette smoking and lung cancer. Even today, people argue, "My grandmother smoked her entire life and died at the ripe old age of 90 from natural causes. How can cigarettes possibly cause cancer?" The reality is that cigarette smoking is only one portion, albeit a big one, of the causal puzzle, that when pieced together leads to lung cancer. This is true of most diseases today. Instead, when physicians talk about cause, they are really talking about risk factors that influence the odds of developing a particular illness. Depression, a complex illness, is more like an illness with multiple causes that influence the odds of someone developing it. Depression runs in families but is not 100% heritable. Depression may occur in someone with no family history for the illness. When considering the causes of depression, the odds are impacted by a variety of sources inside and outside of a person. This variety constitutes what is called the **biopsychosocial** model that is typically employed. In this model, consideration is given to biological, psychological, and social factors that may contribute to the onset of depression. This model influences most diseases of lifestyle. Look at, for instance, heart disease. Applying the biopsychosocial model to heart disease demonstrates biological risk factors of family history, the presence of high blood pressure and high cholesterol, and atherosclerosis; psychological risk factors of type A personality and/or an inability to handle stressful events; and social risk factors of smoking, diet, and activity level.

Biopsychosocial
a model used to describe the possible origins of risk factors for the development of various mental illnesses.

Biologically, depression is associated with changes in various neurotransmitter levels and activity, commonly referred to as a **chemical imbalance** in the brain. Additionally, depression frequently runs in families, suggesting a genetic, or heritable, aspect to the illness. Medical conditions and sometimes the medications used to treat those conditions can also cause depressive symptoms. Psychologically, certain personality types are more prone to developing depression. People who have low self-esteem and a pessimistic outlook are at higher risk for depression. Other psychological disorders, such as anxiety, psychotic, or substance abuse disorders, increase the odds of developing depression. Socially, depression is linked to stressful life events,

Chemical imbalance
a common vernacular for what is thought to be occurring in the brain in patients suffering from mental illness.

usually entailing loss, such as of a spouse, child, job, or financial security. Depression, however, can also be linked to events generally considered to be uplifting rather than stressful, although from the body's reaction, they are stressful. These events can include marriage, the birth of a child, a job change or promotion, or a move to a new neighborhood or home.

9. What chemicals regulate emotions? What chemical imbalance occurs in depression?

Literally thousands of different chemicals participate in brain function and fall into different groups based on their chemical structure, mechanism of action, **psychotropic** effects, where they originally came from, or disease process that they are designed to treat. The chemicals affecting emotional states in the brain consist of three broad types of compounds: neurotransmitters, which are chemically derived from single amino acids, the core constituents of proteins; neuropeptides, small links of amino acids that together form a protein with psychoactive effects; and hormones, chemicals made in different regions throughout the body that are released into the blood stream and have psychoactive effects.

Psychotropic
usually referring to medications that, as a result of their physiological effects on the brain, lead to direct psychological effects.

Biogenic amines
a group of compounds in the nervous system that participate in the regulation of brain activity.

Hundreds of different neurotransmitters exist in the brain, and they fall in different groups as well based on their chemical structure. The **biogenic amines** are the most understood group of neurotransmitters and include dopamine, **serotonin**, and **norepinephrine**. Each biogenic amine is made within a small region of the brain, but axons from the neurons in those areas of the brain disseminate these neurotransmitters widely throughout the brain. All three of the noted biogenic

Serotonin
a neurotransmitter involved in mood regulation, anxiety, pain perception, appetite, sleep, sexual behavior, and impulsive behavior.

Norepinephrine
a neurotransmitter that is involved in the regulation of mood, arousal, and memory.

amines are involved in the regulation of mood. Dopamine, for example, is implicated in the brain's natural reward system and, therefore, is seen as pleasure generating. Norepinephrine is linked to the hormone epinephrine, also known as adrenaline. Adrenaline has become associated with all risk-taking activities that cause a "rush." Serotonin traditionally was linked to activities involving sleep, appetite, and sexual function, better known in psychiatry as vegetative activities, but more recently has been implicated in control of mood and anxiety.

Three neurotransmitters (or chemicals) with a large body of evidence supporting their roles in mood regulation are dopamine, serotonin, and norepinephrine, although ongoing research is investigating the role of various other neurotransmitters in depression as well. Where does the evidence come from? Basically, the evidence stems from three sources: primarily from our understanding of the biological and clinical effects of various psychoactive agents on the brain; secondarily from postmortem human studies; and finally, from experimentation with animal models. Some of the evidence includes the following:

- Depletion of serotonin (by other medications such as certain antihypertensives) can precipitate depression.
- Patients who have successfully committed suicide by violent means have evidence for reduced serotonin levels in the **central nervous system** based on postmortem analyses.
- Antidepressant medications increase the functional capacity of dopamine, serotonin, and norepinephrine to varying degrees in the brain.

Central nervous system
nerve cells and their support cells in the brain and spinal cord.

- Successfully treated depression with an antidepressant can be reversed by blocking transport of the amino acid **tryptophan** used to make serotonin.
- Nearly all effective antidepressant medications affect receptors for dopamine, norepinephrine, and serotonin in the brains of animal models.

Tryptophan
1 of the 20 amino acids that constitute the building blocks of proteins in the body. Tryptophan is the building block for serotonin.

In depression, the biogenic amines are believed to be insufficient in quantity within the synaptic cleft, and thus, proper communication to the receiving neuron does not occur. Medications used as treatment for depression typically improve the signals between nerves by directly increasing the amount of dopamine, serotonin, or norepinephrine activity in the synaptic clefts between nerves. This can be done by blocking either the destruction of the neurotransmitter or the reuptake of the neurotransmitter. There is, however, a secondary effect. Increasing the amount of neurotransmitter in the synaptic cleft affects both the amount of other neurotransmitters as well as the numbers of receptors available to receive these neurotransmitters. If one thinks of the body as continually adjusting itself in order to maintain a proper balance, the increase in the amount of neurotransmitter causes a compensatory decrease in the number of receptors in order to balance out the relationship between the two. This is known in neuroscience as down-regulation. Down-regulation can take approximately 4 to 6 weeks to occur, which is one theory as to the reason that it may take 4 to 6 weeks for an antidepressant to have its full effect. A balance exists between the various chemicals involved in the regulation of signals that effect mood, and therefore, depression can be viewed simply as a chemical imbalance. Balance is therefore restored through the use of medications that either block destruction of the chemicals or block the reuptake of those chemicals. Monoamine oxidase inhibitors (MAOIs) are a class of medications that block the destruction of the chemicals. Other **antidepressants**, including the commonly used serotonin reuptake inhibitors, block the return or transport of serotonin or norepinephrine into the sending neuron so that more of the neurotransmitter remains in the cleft. Some studies have demonstrated evidence of similar brain changes in response to interventions other than medications, such as from psychotherapy, as well. It is important to keep in mind that it is not clear at present whether the "chemical imbalance" is the cause or result of depression as the two appear simultaneously. Therefore the fact that depression can improve with therapy and medication is not surprising and the term "chemical imbalance" does not argue for one approach over another.

Antidepressant
a drug specifically marketed for and capable of relieving the symptoms of clinical depression.

10. What is the difference between psychiatry and psychology?

Historically, the sciences were considered a part of philosophy called natural philosophy, as they pertained to thinkers concerned with the state of nature. Psychology was that part of natural philosophy associated with human nature. As philosophers of human nature were primarily concerned with actions that could be judged as right and wrong, psychology was considered a moral science. This was the purview of philosophers who were contemplating the normal range of human behavior. Alternatively, abnormal behavior, more commonly known as psychopathology, was generally the purview of physicians. Those physicians consisted of either neurologists or general practitioners whose responsibilities included the general medical care of patients committed to asylums for the mentally ill. No special training existed in the diagnosis and treatment of mental illness. Expertise was therefore derived primarily from exposure to those types of patients and not by any specialized training. When science separated from philosophy with the introduction of the experimental method, the field of psychology also began to adopt an equally experimental approach. Psychology retained its status in the university as an academic discipline devoted to understanding how human behavior and the mind worked.

Freud, trained as a neurologist, was the first physician to develop and describe a method of therapy whereby the patient said whatever came to mind—called **free association**. The therapist would listen critically and link various dreams, memories, and stories that the patient related to him or her and provide an interpretation for the patient as to the **unconscious** meanings of the patient's narrative. Through these interpretations, the patient developed insight, allowing the patient to make changes in both his or her attitudes and behavior so that he or she could be relieved of pain and suffering. Freud coined this method psychoanalysis. This was the beginning of modern psychotherapy. Freud was instrumental in expanding the treatment of mental illness in such a way as to take it out of the asylums and put it in the office. He also strongly believed that although psychoanalysis required very specialized training a medical degree was not required in order to learn and practice the technique. Thus, the door was opened to psychologists becoming clinicians rather

Free association

the mental process of saying aloud whatever comes to mind, suppressing the natural tendency to censor or filter thoughts.

Unconscious

an underlying motivation for behavior that is not available to the conscious or thoughtful mind, which has developed over the course of life experience.

than solely scientists and philosophers. Since that time, universities and professional schools of psychology have expanded to train psychologists to become clinicians. Psychology students can choose a career track in either research or the practice of clinical psychology. A clinical psychologist typically has undergone 4 years of undergraduate education and 4 years of graduate education in psychology, followed by a 1-year internship in a mental healthcare setting, treating patients under the supervision of a senior psychologist.

Psychiatrists have a radically different educational path, having grown as a specialty out of the asylum system where physicians took responsibility for the general healthcare of the mentally ill who were confined to asylums. Psychiatrists begin studies in human anatomy and physiology as medical students. Graduating with a medical degree and the same educational background as all physicians, psychiatrists spend a year in an internship that may include psychiatry but must include medicine or some other medical rotation and neurology. After internship one spends an additional 3 years as a resident physician, treating patients in a variety of settings under the supervision of a senior psychiatrist. As physicians, psychiatrists are licensed to prescribe medications just as all physicians are. However, because of their specialty, they develop a singular expertise in using medications to treat mental illness.

PART TWO

Diagnosis

What are the symptoms of depression?

How is depression diagnosed?

What are the different types of depression?

More . . .

11. What are the symptoms of depression?

Anthony's comment:

It is possible that a person wouldn't recognize the symptoms they have in order to seek help. In fact it isn't necessary to recognize these symptoms in order to seek help. Your doctor can help sort out and define for you what might be going on and if it is consistent with depression. Symptoms are not only emotional, but physical as well, with such problems as insomnia, excessive worrying, loss of appetite, change in behaviors/activities, change in bowel patterns, etc. When I'm depressed, I have found that I don't want to be bothered by people and prefer not to associate with people I once considered friends.

The signs and symptoms of depression include the following:

- Sadness or irritability
- A loss of enjoyment of once pleasurable activities
- A loss of energy
- Difficulty concentrating
- **Insomnia** or excessive sleep
- Fatigue
- Unexplained physical complaints (e.g., headache, backache, stomach upset)
- Decreased sex drive
- A change in appetite (increased or reduced)
- Feelings of hopelessness, helplessness, and/or worthlessness
- Suicidal thoughts or attempts

Insomnia

the inability to fall asleep, middle of the night awakening, or early morning awakening.

If these symptoms persist for more than 2 weeks, clinical depression may be present. The greater the number of symptoms present, particularly if associated with sadness or irritability, the more likely depression is present. Suicidal thinking warrants an immediate evaluation, especially if associated with hopelessness. As can be seen from the list, many of the features of depression involve physical symptoms. Depression is not strictly a condition in the mind. Lack of energy and fatigue may make it difficult to get moving or follow through with commitments (work, school, and family). Some people exhibit **psychomotor retardation**—a condition in which the body moves very little and very slowly. Symptoms may change over the course of a day with a worse mood in the morning and a better mood at night or vice versa.

Psychomotor retarded

slowed movement, usually as a result of severe clinical depression.

Because of the multitude of physical symptoms in depression, many patients seen by a primary care health provider for certain physical complaints actually have depression. Certainly a physical evaluation excluding any other medical conditions is warranted, but depression needs to be considered as a possible condition. Many times the clinician does not consider it, or when asked about mood or the possibility of depression being present, some patients may become upset, thinking that their doctor considers their symptoms "all in their head." In fact, depression is a medical condition that causes real physical symptoms. Physical symptoms will get better as the depression is treated.

12. How is depression diagnosed?

Depression is diagnosed as part of a complete psychiatric or other mental health evaluation. The evaluation includes a review of current and past symptoms, psychiatric and medical history, family history, social history, and substance-use history. In addition, there is an assessment of the current **mental status**. Although no tests or procedures are available to diagnose depression, in certain circumstances, tests may be ordered in addition to a request for a physical examination in order to exclude any general medical conditions as a cause for the depression. Depending on the circumstances, the clinician may want to obtain collateral information from family members. Based on the symptoms, history, and mental status, a specific diagnosis can be made. The DSM-IV-TR defines a major depressive episode by the following symptoms:

Mental status
a snapshot portrait of one's cognitive and emotional functioning at a particular point in time.

1. Depressed mood for most of the day, nearly every day
2. A loss of interest or pleasure in activities
3. Significant weight loss (not dieting) or weight gain or change in appetite
4. Feelings of worthlessness or inappropriate guilt
5. Decreased concentration
6. Insomnia or **hypersomnia** (excessive sleep)
7. **Psychomotor agitation** or retardation
8. Fatigue or loss of energy
9. Recurrent thoughts of death or suicidal ideation

Hypersomnia
an inability to stay awake. Oversleeping.

Psychomotor agitation
hyperactive or restless movement. It can be seen in highly anxious states, manic mood states, or intoxicated states.

All of the symptoms need not be present except for at least item 1 or item 2. Additional guidelines are available for clinicians to make a diagnosis of major depression; these consider the number of symptoms present. One feature necessary for a diagnosis is a reduction in functional capacity (academic, occupational, or social). There are other forms of depression in addition to major depression, such as **dysthymic** disorder and **bipolar depression**. Dysthymic disorder is a chronic,

Dysthymic
the presence of chronic, mild depressive symptoms.

Bipolar depression
an episode of depression that occurs in the course of bipolar disorder.

"milder" depression, but it can be quite debilitating because of its chronicity. It is less associated with some of the **neurovegetative** symptoms that characterize major depression. Bipolar depression is the depressed phase of a condition called bipolar disorder, also known as "manic depressive disorder." The features of this depression are the same as in major depression, but the patient has a history of prior manic or **hypomanic** episodes. As part of the evaluation, the clinician screens for a history of **mania**, as this can affect the treatment choices of bipolar depression.

Neurovegetative
that part of the nervous system devoted to vegetative or involuntary processes such as respiration, blood pressure, heart rate, temperature, sleep, appetite, sexual arousal, etc.

Hypomanic
a milder form of mania with the same symptoms but of lesser intensity.

13. What are the different types of depression?

Mania
a condition characterized by elevation of mood associated with racing thoughts, decreased need for sleep, hyperactivity, and poor impulse control.

Several types of depression exist. Depressed (or irritable) mood or a loss of interest in pleasurable activities is characteristic of all types, and all types have to cause impairment in functioning. There are some differences in symptom presentation, however, and treatment approaches may vary somewhat. The different types of depression include the following:

- Major depressive disorder
- Dysthymic disorder
- Seasonal affective disorder
- Bipolar depression
- Depressive disorder not otherwise specified

In major depression, qualifiers can be added to the diagnosis, such as "atypical," "melancholic," or "**postpartum** onset." Such qualifiers describe a specific pattern of symptom presentation. For example, increased appetite, rejection sensitivity, and a sensation of heaviness of the limbs characterize an atypical major depressive episode. Melancholic depression is most

Postpartum
referring to events occurring within a specified time after giving birth. Usually within the first 4 weeks.

associated with sleep and appetite loss and psychomotor retardation. It also is characterized by a phenomenon known as a **diurnal variation** of mood—feeling much worse in the morning with some improvement in mood by evening.

Diurnal variation

a variation in mood that occurs within a day.

Major depression and dysthymic disorder are the most common forms of depression. Dysthymic disorder is more chronic with persistent sadness nearly daily for at least 2 years. In seasonal affective disorder, the depressive symptoms are the same as in major depression but occur exclusively within one season (usually the winter). Bipolar depression is the depressed phase of a condition called bipolar disorder (discussed later here). In many cases, the symptom presentation of depression does not fit the criteria as described in the DSM-IV-TR. Symptoms, however, may be causing impairment in functioning. The diagnosis of depressive disorder not otherwise specified can be used in those cases. Although the type of depression informs as to prognosis and best treatment modality, in general, all types respond to both medication therapy and talk therapy.

14. Are any blood tests or other tests available for depression?

No objective tests are available for depression. Some tests used in research protocols examine levels of certain stress hormones or look at brain functioning. These are research based only, however, and have no utility in clinical practice. Your doctor may order blood tests to check for any underlying conditions that may mimic depression such as low thyroid hormone. Blood tests or electrocardiograms may be ordered for baseline purposes, depending on the medication that is to be prescribed, as some medications may have effects on certain organ systems in the body.

Although not a required part of an evaluation, some clinicians will use various rating scales and self-report forms to assist in the evaluation process. Scales may be useful in tracking the progression of the depression in a quantifiable way. Comprehensive diagnostic scales can guide the clinician in going through a differential diagnostic process in order to exclude other causes for the symptoms before establishing a diagnosis. Such scales may indeed establish a diagnosis of a depression, but they are based on the same clinical criteria used without a scale. These scales are mostly useful in research to establish reliability in diagnosis and to increase the validity of the study.

15. How do I know whether I have depression versus a "normal" reaction to a problem in my life?

Life events that are stressful can result in normal sadness as well as other symptoms similar to those present during a depressive episode. These symptoms may only last a few days. In the case of **bereavement**, symptoms may last much longer. Bereavement, however, is a normal process. The duration of bereavement can vary between cultural groups. If, however, symptoms begin to prevent an individual from functioning socially or occupationally and academically and persist beyond a couple of months, especially if suicidal thinking is present, then the possibility of a depressive episode being present is much greater. An assessment by a

Bereavement
the period of time spent in mourning for the death of a loved one.

Table 1 Differentiating Depression from Normal Sadness

Increased intensity of symptoms
Increased length of symptoms
No change in mood with changes in external events
Decreased functioning at work/school/home

mental health practitioner would be warranted in such circumstances. Table 1 outlines features that may help differentiate depression from normal sadness.

Although depression has a biological basis, stressful life events often trigger its onset. Certain life events are considered more stressful than others. Divorce, death of a spouse, and death of a child are considered very stressful. Additional stressors include marital arguments, a new job, the presence of a serious personal illness, going to college, moving, marriage, and the birth of a child. Sometimes the accumulation of several mild stressors triggers a depressive episode. At one time, it was presumed that there were two types of depression: endogenous (triggered from within, or "biological") or exogenous (triggered from environmental circumstances). Such a distinction is generally not considered applicable anymore, as most depressions are triggered by environmental circumstances, and are likely dependent on the person's genetic vulnerability. A comprehensive mental health evaluation typically identifies social stressors associated with the depression. Depending on the nature of the stressors, different treatment modalities may even be recommended (e.g., family therapy, couples counseling, group therapy).

Again, one of the reasons that so many people do not get treated for depression is because of the belief that the depression may be a normal reaction to a given situation. Sadness is a normal emotion and a normal reaction to many situations, but depression is a condition that adversely affects the entire body; left untreated, it can have significant consequences for the affected individual. Sleep and appetite are adversely affected. The body may have reduced ability to fight infection. Depression can make recovery from stroke or heart attack more difficult. A greater risk exists for drug and alcohol abuse, which in turn can worsen depression and further impair functioning. Because of the risks of untreated depression, it is best to seek mental health consultation if there is any question of the possibility of depression.

16. I have a good job and a loving family. How can I feel depressed?

Anthony's comment:

It seems it would make sense to examine your daily routines to see if indeed problems do exist. It is also important to be evaluated for a medical condition as a cause of the depression. Psychiatrists routinely consider the possibility of medical conditions as a cause, and may recommend a medical workup. I have often been surprised myself when I learn about a famous person for example, who admits to having taken antidepressants, who seems to me to "have it all." I may even wonder, "what's your problem?" when in fact what this shows is that what appears on the surface to be an admirable life, often has many other unknown aspects to it.

As noted previously here, depression is not a condition that depends solely on a person's life circumstances.

Certainly, stressful situations such as loss of job, family problems, or relationship difficulties can trigger the onset of a depressive episode. However, a lack of obvious stressful circumstances does not make a person invulnerable to becoming depressed. This can make it difficult sometimes for others to understand, as they may think, "What do you have to be depressed about?" The depression may be viewed as a lack of personal willpower. You may feel guilty about being unhappy, and again, the idea of needing to "pull myself together" becomes part of your thinking. These thought patterns may impede initiation of treatment. With that said, sometimes when there are no obvious external stressors present, there may be "internal" ones. Perhaps you feel like a failure for not having reached certain goals. Perhaps an unrelated event has triggered fears and anxieties that now fuel a depressive episode. These are potential avenues to be explored in a therapy, to help with **recovery**, and to maintain **remission**.

Recovery
the term used after a time period of 6 months symptom free after successful treatment for a mental illness.

Remission
complete cessation of all symptoms associated with a specific mental illness within the first 6 months of treatment.

17. Are there medical conditions that could be cause for my depression?

Many medical conditions can have depression associated with them, ranging from endocrine (**hormonal**) disorders, cardiac conditions, cancers, vitamin deficiencies, etc. Most often, depression occurs independent of another medical disorder, but if physical signs and symptoms exist other than those typically found in depression, a medical/physical examination to exclude physical causes for depression is warranted. Because of their medical background, psychiatrists routinely consider medical conditions as possible causes for depression and thus will assess a person's medical history. Your psychiatrist may consider obtaining laboratory

Hormonal
referring to the chemicals that are secreted by the endocrine glands and act throughout the body.

tests as part of screening for medical conditions or may defer this evaluation to your primary care physician. If a medical condition exists, it may be difficult to determine with certainty whether the depression is physiologically related or merely co-occurring with the illness. Treatment of the medical disorder may or may not result in resolution of the depression, but resolution of the depression would support the physiologic connection. Even if so connected, it is possible that treatment for depression will still also be needed. Depression can have adverse effects on the body and its recovery from illness; thus, it is very important to treat co-existing depression vigorously. For example, postrecovery cardiac patients do more poorly when depressed, and thus, depression is usually treated more vigorously now in this population than it had been in years past (see Table 2 for a list of some medical conditions that can be associated with depression).

More often, depression worsens existing medical conditions or is the cause itself for physical symptoms. Depression and anxiety can be associated with several physical ailments for which there are no physical cause associated with them. Sometimes, a symptomatic person does not endorse depressed mood, or there is

Table 2 Differentiating Depression from Medical Problems

Endocrine- hyper/hypothyroid, Cushing's disease, Addison's disease, diabetes
Infection- AIDS, Lyme's disease, hepatitis
Cancer- pancreatic, occult, brain
Neurological- dementia, Parkinson's disease, stroke
Cardiac- coronary artery disease, heart failure, heart attack
Medications- antihypertensives, steroids, oral contraceptives

denial of a depressed or anxious mood (perhaps because of negative associations with the idea of mental illness). Instead, the emotional distress is expressed through physical symptoms. Such persons may see many different doctors seeking a "medical" cause of their symptoms. Missing a **mood disorder** in such cases can result in an overuse of healthcare services—not to mention persistent morbidity and decreased productivity in the person. Afflicted persons often show improvement in the physical symptoms with an antidepressant or therapy.

Mood disorder

a type of mental illness that affects mood primarily and cognition secondarily.

18. Why did my doctor diagnose depression when I do not feel depressed?

Anthony's comment:

Daily activities may be stagnated. When a medical specialist met with me for an unrelated condition, and asked about my daily routine, he noted that I must be depressed based on what I told him. I considered this very observant and insightful on the part of my endocrinologist. Depression is not always experienced by a person as strictly an emotional state. My behavior is consistent with depression, even if I am not always cognizant of it. Looking back at what has happened to me in the past couple months, and the pattern of my daily activities, it is clear to me that I have become depressed again.

Part of the misunderstanding that creates so much guilt and shame around clinical depression comes from the fact that many people mistake depression as a symptom for depression as a disease. It is perfectly normal for people to feel sad, to have the "blues," or to feel in a "funk" at times. Life is filled with small and large disappointments and losses. These events are part of the inevitable course of everyone's life history. Therefore, because such feelings are normal, becoming incapacitated by them while others seem to bounce back and move on can inevitably lead one to feelings of guilt and shame for not being "strong enough" to handle seemingly everyday events. One might work extra hard to fight the incapacitating feelings and to avoid either admitting having them or giving into them. When one does, the shame can become so overwhelming that it leads to further denial, withdrawal, or worse, suicidal acts.

There are many times then when the only thing to do is to simply deny feeling depressed. The denial of such feelings can become locked away in one's unconscious in order to prevent perceived harm. Identifying how one feels sometimes becomes as difficult as describing the nose on one's face without ever looking in a mirror. Thus, family and friends may have a better sense of a person's moods or behavior than the person who is depressed. The denial of feelings is not always unconscious. Sometimes people knowingly deny how they feel because they identify it as a sign of moral weakness rather than an illness, or people are so caught up in external events that they have lost sight of how they feel about them. In all of these ways people are not always in touch with the way they feel or behave.

However, clinical depression manifests itself regardless of whether people consciously deny it, are unconsciously unaware that they are feeling sad or depressed, or are so caught up in events that they have lost sight of their feelings. It is important to understand that clinical depression represents a constellation of symptoms that occur simultaneously and not by the simple fact that one feels sad. One should think of clinical depression in the more general physiologic or economic sense of a reduction in activity rather than a feeling of sadness. These symptoms are attributed to a variety of physiological states that are depressed (or slowed down). Thinking is slowed so that concentration and short-term memory are impacted. Interest in activities slows to a standstill, leading to a lack of motivation to do anything but the most basic tasks. Appetite is slowed so that people often lose their sense of hunger, taste, or interest in food. This can paradoxically lead to weight gain, as food is chosen that is the most immediately rewarding, usually high in fats and carbohydrates. Bowels slow, leading to indigestion and constipation. Energy slows, causing feelings of fatigue. Sleep slows, leading to disruption. All of these physiologic states are reduced or depressed in a broad sense independently of whether one feels sad, although as a result the person will admit to a loss of interest in activities that he or she previously enjoyed.

Thus, there are times when a doctor diagnoses depression in the absence of feeling sad or depressed. Some populations or age groups are more susceptible to depression in the absence of feeling sad. For example, some cultures do not have language to describe feelings, and instead, feelings are identified **somatically**, through bodily complaints. As people age, their ability to identify their feelings diminishes as well. Often, older people become so preoccupied with their bodily functions that they lose sight of the impact that their physical complaints are having on them. Under these

Somatic

referring to the body. Somatic therapy refers to all treatments that have direct physiological effects.

circumstances, patients often come to see a psychiatrist as much out of frustration with their internist as clinical need. They often report no feelings of depression whatsoever but complain bitterly about how their physical complaints are preventing them from doing all of the activities that normally gave them pleasure in life. They often report that they can no longer garden, golf, read, do crossword puzzles, or follow the news because they are so consumed with worry about their physical condition. These are situations in which depression may be diagnosed in the absence of subjective feelings of depression.

19. What is bipolar disorder?

Individuals with bipolar disorder classically have cycles of depression alternating with euphoric/irritable mood states (called mania). There are several disorders of mood in addition to the depressive disorders listed in Question 13 that involve depression as well as manic or hypomanic mood states. The additional mood disorders are as follows:

- Bipolar I disorder
- Bipolar II disorder
- Cyclothymia
- Mood disorder not otherwise specified

A manic episode is defined as a period of euphoric and/or irritable mood that lasts at least 4 days; it is characterized by a decreased need for sleep, racing thoughts, the need to keep speaking, inflated self-esteem or grandiose thinking, and excess goal-directed activities. The same group of symptoms also defines a hypomanic episode, but the severity is judged to be less. Individuals in the midst of a manic episode can become psychotic and require hospitalization.

In bipolar I disorder, the person must have a history of at least one manic episode. The number of depressive episodes can be as few as none to any amount. Classically, an afflicted person alternates between episodes with normal mood in between. However, cycles can consist of any frequency of mood states in any order. Bipolar II disorder is comprised of depressive episodes alternating with hypomanic episodes only (no mania). In cyclothymia, no major depressive episode has occurred, but mild depressive episodes alternate with hypomanic states. Mood disorder not otherwise specified is also a condition of exclusion in that a mood disorder is considered present, but the criteria have not been met for the other conditions in the DSM-IV-TR. In someone presenting with depression, these conditions can only be excluded by a thorough history of symptoms and episodes in the past. Sometimes the patient does not recall such episodes, however, such that a bipolar condition is not learned of until the treatment for depression is initiated.

20. My husband is depressed and has mood swings. Is he a manic depressive?

Mood swings are often thought to be synonymous with having manic depression. The presence of "mood swings," however, is not enough to determine that a person is manic depressive. Many depressed persons can have ups and downs in their mood. The distinction is important because manic depression is another name for a condition called bipolar disorder (see Question 19), and depression in bipolar disorder is treated differently than in major depression. Bipolar disorder is less frequent than major depressive disorder, occurring in approximately 1% of the population. It is also more closely associated with family history and, in general, is a more severe illness. Bipolar depression differs from major depression in that the individual has to have experienced at least one manic or hypomanic episode in his or her lifetime. Although experiencing mania or hypomania is often referred to as having "mood swings," there are specific criteria to define these mood states. Mood swings can mean many things to many people—from constant crying to episodes of irritability or anger. Recent research has also determined that the symptoms accompanying major depressive disorder may vary dramatically over time. Such variability can be misinterpreted as "mood swings." Manic or hypomanic episodes are strictly characterized by a decreased need for sleep (not the same as insomnia), inflated self-esteem (**grandiosity**), rapid and **pressured speech** (the need to keep talking), euphoric mood, and increased activity level. Duration criteria are required to make the diagnosis as well. It is important that the strict criteria are used because depression alone can be a cause for irritability and anger management problems, both of which can look like mood swings. Once it is determined that a manic or hypomanic episode has occurred in the past, then the diagnosis must reflect that, as the treatment approach may be different and different risks are associated with taking antidepressants.

Grandiosity
the tendency to consider the self or one's ideas better or more superior to what is reality.

Pressured speech
characterized by the need to keep speaking.

21. I became irritable and agitated on my antidepressant. My doctor thinks that I have become "hypomanic." What does that mean?

Manic depressive disorder, or bipolar disorder, can only be diagnosed if someone has a history of at least one manic (bipolar I) or hypomanic (bipolar II) episode. Sometimes, a person's first episode of a mood disorder is that of depression; therefore, a possibility exists of a depressed individual really having bipolar disorder. The likelihood of this occurring increases if there is a family history of bipolar disorder. If a person with depression actually has bipolar disorder, an antidepressant may trigger the onset of a hypomanic or manic mood state. This is why bipolar depressed persons usually require a **mood stabilizer** when taking an antidepressant.

Mood stabilizer typically refers to medications for the treatment and prevention of mood swings, such as from depression to mania.

Becoming hypomanic or even manic on an antidepressant, however, is not diagnostic of bipolar disorder. These reactions can occur in nonbipolar depressed persons. If you have a manic response, your doctor will want to stop the antidepressant. Further inquiry into past personal and family history will be done to be sure that evidence of past hypomanic or manic episodes was not missed. Once the antidepressant is stopped, your hypomanic or manic symptoms should resolve. If they do not, then bipolar disorder is likely present. If resolved, another antidepressant can be tried, as the manic response will not necessarily occur with another medication. If it does occur again, then a mood stabilizer may be necessary in conjunction with an antidepressant.

22. I have been diagnosed with a mild depression. Does that mean a quicker recovery?

Several types of depression exist. Each is characterized by a specified symptom presentation. The most common types of depression are major depressive disorder, dysthymic disorder, and bipolar depression. Major depressive disorder is given a qualifier of mild, moderate, or severe, depending on the number of symptoms. In a mild major depression, treatment is essentially the same as for a moderate to severe depression, but the **response** to the treatment may not necessarily be better. Certainly, the required interventions may not be as intense as those used for a severe depression (e.g., hospitalization or twice a week or more therapy). Dysthymic disorder is also considered a mild type of depression, but its course is more apt to be chronic; thus, recovery may be more difficult than for someone who has a discrete episode of major depression. In particular, some individuals with dysthymia have a major depressive episode as well (called "**double depression**"), which may complicate the treatment. Although dysthymia is not associated with the same degree of morbidity and mortality as major depression, it does cause functional impairment and thus affects a person's well-being. Dysthymic disorder is generally treated the same as a major depression, but again, treatment interventions may not need to be as intense, depending on the level of functional impairment. For example, hospitalization is not likely necessary for dysthymic disorder. In terms of time to recovery, it typically takes 4 to 6 weeks for depression to go into remission once medication therapy is initiated. It may take longer if psy-

Response

referring to at least a 50% reduction but not complete cessation of all symptoms associated with a specific mental illness.

Double depression

the co-occurrence of a major depressive episode with dysthymic disorder.

chotherapy is the only intervention. The type of depression present does not signify the likelihood of response to treatment, although it may inform as to prognosis. For example, bipolar depression may require longer maintenance treatment than one episode of major depression.

23. I have been diagnosed with depression. What do I tell my family and friends?

Anne's comment:

Because of the stigma surrounding depression, we have been careful with whom we share the facts of what we are dealing with. It has been essential to have the support of family members, and we have found it extremely important that the family members living in the household with the depressed individual work with a therapist so that they can have a comprehensive understanding of depression and be a part of the healing process.

Anthony's comment:

I have preferred not to discuss my struggle with depression with friends or family. I have found that family members may become needlessly frightened, and friends are more apt to shrug it off with comments like "who isn't depressed?" or "you're just stressed out." Be careful in whom you decide to share with. In spite of extensive media coverage of depression, there remain doubts about depression and what it is about. People may not give you the reaction that you want, which can cause further problems as well, as you may question the sincerity of your friendships. Unless in borderline need of hospitalization, it may be better not to say anything, depending on the situation.

Although there is a greater understanding in society about depression, stigmatization continues to exist, and there can be concern about what to share about the condition with your family and friends. The decision as to sharing information about your diagnosis can be fraught with more worries as to how others will perceive you than, for example, if you had to inform them of an infectious disease, a heart condition, diabetes, or even cancer. As with any other illness, you have a right to your privacy in terms of disclosure. Certainly, the more you can open up about your depression, as with any illness, to people close to you, the more support you can garnish in your time of need. It is reasonable to use discretion in sharing anything personal about yourself; the same holds true regarding your depression. If you do not discuss it with people closest to you, you may be more apt to feel shame about it and inhibited in obtaining help and remaining on the treatment plan that you need. Stigmatization results when people hide shamefully behind what ails them. It is easier for people to hold on to their biases if they believe that they do not know anyone with depression or any other mental illness. Close family and friends are more apt to be supportive than you may believe. Question 92 addresses the issue on family involvement further.

24. Who is qualified to diagnose and treat depression?

Many clinicians of various educational backgrounds are qualified to diagnose and treat depression. The choice of practitioner type in part will depend on need for therapy, medication, or both. Your internist or family practice doctor can diagnose and treat depression, as can a nurse practitioner. They may wish to refer you to a mental health specialist, however, if therapy is needed or if a more in-depth evaluation is warranted.

Most insurance plans have participants who can provide mental health services, although sometimes the choices available on a given plan are limited. Geographic location also may dictate choice of practitioner, as shortages of certain clinicians exist in some areas of the United States (e.g., child and adolescent psychiatrists). Mental health specialists who can evaluate for and treat depression include the following:

- Social workers
- Psychologists
- Psychiatric nurse specialists
- Psychiatrists

In seeking a mental health specialist, it is important to choose someone with proper credentials and training. Anyone can call himself or herself a psychotherapist without having specialized training or a degree. It is appropriate to ask the therapist about his or her training and background in the assessment and treatment of depression. Credentials for the previously noted mental health specialists follow.

Social workers provide a full range of mental health services, including assessment, diagnosis, and treatment. They have completed undergraduate work in social work or other fields, followed by postgraduate education to obtain a Masters of Social Work (MSW) or a doctorate degree. An MSW is required in order to practice as a clinical social worker or to provide therapy. Most states require practicing social workers to be licensed, certified, or registered. Postgraduate education is 2 years with courses in social welfare, psychology, family systems, child development, diagnosis, and child and elder abuse/neglect. During the 2 years of coursework, social work students participate in internships concordant with their interest. After completion of the master's program, direct clinical supervision is usually required for a period of time to apply for a license, which may vary from state to state.

Psychologists have completed undergraduate work followed by several years of postgraduate studies in order to receive a doctorate degree (PhD or PsyD) in psychology. Graduate psychology education includes study of a variety of subjects, notably statistics, social psychology, developmental psychology, personality theory, psychological testing (paper and pencil tests to help assess personality characteristics, intelligence, learning difficulties, and evidence of psychopathology), psychotherapeutic techniques, history and philosophy of psychology, and psychopharmacology and physiological psychology. After the coursework, a year is spent in a mental health setting providing psychotherapeutic care and psychological testing under the supervision of a senior psychologist. Psychologists must demonstrate a minimum number of hours (usually approximately 1,500) before eligibility to sit for state psychology licensure exams.

Psychiatric nurse specialists have completed undergraduate work, typically in nursing, and have obtained postgraduate education in nursing at the master's or doctorate level. Master's programs are 2 years with coursework consisting of study in physiology, pathophysiology, psychopathology, pharmacology, **psychosocial** and psychotherapeutic treatment modalities, advanced nursing, and diagnosis. The training includes clinical work under supervision. Licensing varies from state to state.

Psychosocial

pertaining to environmental circumstances that can impact one's psychological well-being.

Psychiatrists are medical doctors with specialized training in psychiatry. They have completed undergraduate work followed by 4 years of medical school. Medical education is grounded in basic sciences of anatomy, physiology, pharmacology, microbiology, histology, immunology, and pathology, followed by 2 years of clinical rotations through specialties that include medicine, surgery, pediatrics, obstetrics and gynecology, family practice, and psychiatry (as well as other elective clerkships). During this time, medical students must pass two examinations toward licensure. After graduation from medical school, physicians have a year of internship that may include at least 4 months in a primary care specialty such as medicine or pediatrics and 2 months of neurology. After internship, physicians must take and pass a third exam toward licensure in order to be eligible for licensure (and subsequently practice) in any state. Psychiatrists in training have 3 more years of specialty training in residency, the successful completion of which makes them eligible for board certification. After residency, many psychiatrists pursue further training in a fellowship that can last an additional 2 years. Such fellowships include child and adolescent psychiatry, geriatric psychiatry, consultation–liaison psychiatry, addiction psychiatry, forensic psychiatry, and research. To become board certified, psychiatrists take both written and oral examinations. Certain psychiatry specialties also have a board certification process. Board certification is not a requirement to practice and may not be obtained immediately after completion of residency, although many hospitals and insurance companies do require physicians to be board certified within a specified number of years in order to treat patients in their facility or receive reimbursement.

In addition to seeking a private practitioner for mental health services, different types of facilities/programs are available to obtain an evaluation and treatment, in which various mental health specialists work, including community mental health centers, hospital psychiatry departments and outpatient clinics, university-affiliated programs, social service agencies, and employee-assistance programs.

PART THREE

Risk/ Prevention/ Epidemiology

What are the risk factors associated with depression?

Are certain people more susceptible to depression?

I have recently been diagnosed with depression. What are the risks that my children will inherit it?

More . . .

25. What are the risk factors associated with depression?

The concept of risk is a modern one. The word derives from the Italian *riscare*, meaning "to dare." Before such a concept, the future could only be predicted by consulting the gods, prophets, or astrologers, and when bad things happened, they were attributed to fate. The concept of risk was born out of a simple yet practical question regarding games of chance when money was at stake. Given certain known events that just occurred in the game, what are the odds for winning the game? From there, everything about predicting the future grew and forecasting with degrees of certainty for future events of all kinds developed. Knowledge of risk gives one some power over future events so as to make the odds more favorable to one's goals. For example, although wearing seat belts does not change the odds of getting into an accident, it does change the odds of surviving one. In medicine, the knowledge of risk factors helps to understand the odds of developing certain diseases. It is important, however, to remember that odds, no matter how favorable or unfavorable, are still just odds with the outcome for any particular event still unknown. Just because the odds of developing lung cancer are greater for one who smokes a pack of cigarettes a day than one who does not does not mean that the outcomes are certain.

There are risk factors that one can change and risk factors that one cannot. One cannot change the genes inherited from one's parents, but one can use the knowledge of one's family history to help make choices in life to reduce other risk factors contributing to the probability of developing a particular disease. Thus, recommendations for various diagnostic tests for breast cancer, colon cancer, and heart disease vary depending on whether someone has a family history for a particular condition. With all of this in mind, the risk factors for depression are as follows:

- Gender: Depression is two times more likely in females.
- Age: The peak age of onset is 20–40 years.
- Family history: A person is at one and a half to three times higher risk when he or she has a positive family history for mood disorders.
- Marital status: Separated and divorced persons report higher rates. Married males have lower rates than unmarried males, and married females have higher rates than unmarried females.
- Postpartum: There is an increased risk for the 6-month period after childbirth.
- Negative life events: A possible association exists.
- Early parental death: A possible association exists.
- Premorbid personality factors: A possible association exists.
- Co-morbid psychiatric illnesses: A clear association exists.
- Substance abuse or alcoholism history: A clear association exists.
- Socioeconomic status: A possible association exists.
- Childhood conduct and behavior problems: There is a 20% increase at the age of 21 years.

The risk factors of developing recurrent depression are as follows:

- Multiple prior episodes
- Incomplete recoveries from prior episodes

- A severe episode
- A chronic episode
- Bipolar or psychotic features

In depression, the risk factors that one has control over are very limited when compared with diseases such as heart disease that has opportunities for lowering cholesterol, blood pressure, and weight, through various options, including diet, exercise, smoking cessation, and prescription medications. It is often difficult, if not impossible, to change exposure to any of the risk factors for depression mentioned previously here, except for substance abuse and alcoholism, and yet the perceived level of control over developing depression is much greater than other diseases, another paradox of mental illness! Regarding the risk of **recurrence**, some control over risk factors can be taken by ensuring aggressive treatment with a competent clinician or team of clinicians and sticking to the treatment plan, with frequent follow-up visits to ensure that the symptoms are controlled effectively with all available therapies.

Recurrence

the return of symptoms of a mental illness after complete recovery, considered to have occurred after a period of 6 months symptom free.

26. Are certain people more susceptible to depression?

Women are clearly at greater risk for developing depression than men. This may be due to two factors. First, women are physiologically different, which may explain some of the variance. More importantly, women are psychologically different, and this psychology is shaped by both their different physiology and also by the different cultural expectations placed on them. They are expected to express their feelings more, and it is more socially acceptable for them to admit to being depressed, although formal studies have demonstrated that men and women are equally likely to report their depressive symptoms. Depression often leads to withdrawal, which can be interpreted as passivity in women, also more acceptable in Western culture. Withdrawal in men is generally interpreted as a sign of weakness, and thus, the men who withdraw usually describe it as a choice without any change in mood. Thus, it is interpreted more as an independent act and is recharacterized in more socially acceptable terms such as stoicism. Social factors likely play a large roll in the higher rates of depression in women as well (see Question 80).

Certain ethnic groups are more susceptible. A correlation appears to exist between latitude and susceptibility to depression. Northern Europeans are the most susceptible, with Scandinavians suffering from the highest rates and Mediterraneans suffering from the lowest rates. Certain races also appear to be more susceptible, with whites suffering greater rates than blacks. Recently, a cultural shift has occurred in Japan as a result of the introduction of safe and effective antidepressants used to treat milder forms of depression. As Buddhism has heavily influenced Japanese society, the notion that life is filled primarily with suffering has been the accepted paradigm. In contrast, Western culture tends to be more positive and hopeful. Thus, feeling sad about one's lot in life in Japan was considered the norm, whereas in Western culture, it is considered abnormal. As Japan has become more Westernized and Buddhism less valued, the notion of milder forms of depression that are effectively treated with antidepressant medications has become more accepted.

Obesity plays a role in the development of depression, counteracting the myth of Falstaff or "Jolly Old St. Nick." Studies are beginning to demonstrate that significant weight loss in patients with clinical obesity can lead to those patients being able to come off of antidepressants along with other medications. Depression appears to be linked with obesity in a manner similar to hypertension, heart disease, sleep apnea, joint pain, and diabetes. There may be some correlation with obesity, being female, and suffering higher rates of depression. Females have, on average, higher percentages of body fat than males, and body fat has higher estrogen levels, the hormone involved in female development.

Certain personality styles are more susceptible to depression, with shy, reserved, or dependent people being at higher risk than outgoing, sociable, or independent people. This is truer for males than females, again because being shy, reserved, or dependent is more culturally acceptable in females than males. Body fat and personality style have a significant biological basis, although both are clearly shaped by environmental factors.

27. I have recently been diagnosed with depression. What are the risks that my children will inherit it?

Anne's comment:

My husband has suffered from depression much of his adult life and has a history of depression in his family. We watched our children closely, as we were concerned about the possibility of an inherited predisposition to the illness. To date, two of our four children have been diagnosed with and are being treated for bipolar disorder.

Many different studies have been conducted to examine the influence of genetics on the development of depression. **First-degree relatives** of persons with major depression are two to three times more likely to have major depression than are the first-degree relatives of nondepressed persons. In **adoption studies**, the biological children of affected (depressed) parents remain at an increased risk for a mood disorder even when adopted by nonaffected (nondepressed) parents. Identical twins (who share 100% of genetic material) have **concordance** rates for depression of approximately 50%, and nonidentical twins have concordance rates of 10% to 25%. In a strictly genetic illness, identical twins would both be affected because they share 100% of the genes. Twin studies have shown that a twin of a depressed person has only a 50% likelihood of also having depression. This number, however, is significantly greater than the rate in nonidentical twins, thereby demonstrating that there is at least some genetic contribution to development of this disorder. The fact that there is not 100% concordance between identical twins demonstrates that environmental influences also have a role in precipitating a depressive episode.

First-degree relative
immediate biologically related family member, such as biological parents or full siblings.

Adoption study
a scientific study designed to control for genetic relatedness and environmental influences by comparing siblings adopted into different families.

Concordance
in genetics, a similarity in a twin pair with respect to presence of absence of illness.

Life circumstances are often expected to precipitate a depressive episode in affected individuals. Trauma, financial distress, death of a loved one, and relationship problems are some types of stressors that may be associated with development of depression. No matter how extreme, however, no specific environmental situation will cause a depressive episode in all persons. Therefore, environmental conditions alone are not usually sufficient to explain a depression. The specific event more typically will precipitate a depression in one who is vulnerable to its development at that time.

Putting together genetic and environmental factors as contributors to the onset of depression means that with a family history of depression, an individual has a higher **relative risk** than the general population for developing depression. In fact, the greater number of mood disorders that are present in a person's family, the higher the risk becomes for development of depression. Stressful life events, specific environmental circumstances, or certain psychological processes may serve as a trigger of a depressive episode in someone with a genetic predisposition for the disorder.

Relative risk
a ratio of incidence of a disorder in persons exposed to a risk factor to the incidence of a disorder in persons not exposed to the same risk factor.

28. Is there a link between childhood abuse and depression?

Being a victim of child abuse places one at significant risk for adult depression. Studies have found that a majority of young adults who experienced abuse in childhood have had at least one psychiatric disorder diagnosed at the age of 21 years. The biopsychosocial model can be used to illustrate the elevated risk. Biologically, many victims of child abuse have family histories of mental illness and depression, which alone can predispose someone for adult depression. Also, childhood abuse can result in physical injury to the brain. In addition to poor physical health, studies have shown evidence for impaired brain development secondary to abuse and neglect. Such brain damage can result from direct effects (e.g., shaken baby syndrome) or from the effects of stress on the brain secondary to the **hyperarousal** that children experience when chronically abused.

Hyperarousal
a heightened state of alertness to external and internal stimuli.

Psychologically, the consequences of abuse can include low self-esteem, depression, and relationship difficulties. Suffering from child abuse may result in the development of a "**learned helplessness**" style of coping. Learned helplessness is a concept that developed out of the principles of classical (or **Pavlovian**) conditioning. **Classical conditioning** is a form of learning that occurs when a stimulus is paired in time with a reward that causes a response in the subject. Pavlov, a Russian physiologist, who used dogs as his subjects, conducted the basic experiments. In the experiment, a bell (stimulus) is paired with food (reward), causing the dog to salivate. After repeated pairings, the food could be removed, and the bell alone would cause the dog to salivate. In a similar experiment, a bell is paired with an electrical shock, causing the dog to jump to a safe area. After repeated pairings, the bell alone would signal the dog to jump to the safe area, thus avoiding the shock. However, suppose there is no safe area to jump to? After a while, the dog stops jumping, as there is no way to avoid the shock. This behavior is often accompanied by physiologic changes that mimic depression with the dog losing energy, appetite, and sleep. Even after a safe area is returned, the dog does not respond and take advantage of it because it has learned to believe that there is nothing that it can do to avoid the shock. Several human experiments have firmly established this as a phenomenon in humans as well. Feelings of helplessness are quickly established, and the generalization of these feelings to other situations can take over, making one also feel a sense of hopelessness, a feeling of wanting to give up, and a general loss of interest. The paradigm of learned helplessness fits perfectly with victims of child abuse. They are small and vulnerable. They are in the seemingly most protected environment of their lives, and it is filled with unpredictable threats with no possibility of

Learned helplessness
a behavioral pattern that occurs after repeated exposure to noxious stimuli that is characterized by withdrawal, passivity, and reduced activity level.

Pavlovian
from the discoverer Ivan Pavlov, the method of learning known as classical conditioning.

Classical conditioning
a type of learning that results when a conditioned and an unconditioned stimulus is associated, resulting in a similar response to both stimuli (see Pavlovian).

escape. Additionally, they feel guilty that they are the cause of the abuse, further damaging their self-esteem and sense of hopefulness.

From a social standpoint, the likelihood of being a victim of child abuse increases dramatically in children born of young unwed mothers with little economic means and in those who suffer from depression. Most unwed mothers struggle with supporting their families and find themselves economically challenged between having to go on welfare to spend time raising their children or working at minimum wage jobs and risking neglecting their children. Under these circumstances, many women attach themselves to men whose investment in their children is significantly reduced because of their lack of genetic relatedness. The costs of raising children are far less likely to be tolerated by parents who are not invested in their children. Numerous studies of child abuse cross-culturally have demonstrated that the rates of child abuse dramatically increase with the presence of a stepparent.

Not all abused children will experience long-term consequences, however. Factors that affect long-term consequences include the child's age and stage of development when the abuse occurred; the type of abuse; the frequency, duration, and severity of abuse; and the relationship between abuser and victim. There may be protective factors that improve long-term outcomes in abused children as well. These include resilience factors such as high intelligence and optimism in the child, access to social supports, and access to healthcare.

29. A family member has depression. Is there anything I can do to help?

Anne's comment:

In addition to all of the excellent points made by the authors in response to this question, the small daily gestures of support are so important. Being patient, not taking irritable behavior to heart, maintaining a positive attitude instead of mirroring a negative one, and seeking therapy for yourself when you feel overwhelmed by the demands of caring for your sick partner or child are things you can do to create a healing environment. All family members living with a depressed person are affected in some manner, and it helps to recognize the effects and address them with professional guidance.

Anthony's comment:

1) Listen, 2) contact the proper mental health professional, and 3) stay with your family member if you think he or she is suicidal. You may have to step away from the situation for awhile once you have gone through these three steps, because ultimately, as with any medical condition, your family member will need to seek assistance on his or her own.

Helping your family member seek treatment is one of the more important ways to assist. Many individuals have difficulty taking the first step of making an appointment with a mental health practitioner. If the person is already in treatment, helping him or her remember the appointments and providing encouragement to stay in the treatment will be of tremendous help. Accompanying your family member to any appointments to provide feedback to the clinician can be of help, as some depressed persons have difficulty noting either improvements or setbacks in their condition. If on medication, assistance and reminders to take medication are useful, as a lack in **compliance** with medication is a common reason for **relapse**. If there is reason to believe that someone is suicidal, it is critical to seek assistance as soon as possible. If a depressed family member refuses to get assistance, it is prudent to call the local authorities, such as emergency medical services, to have the individual evaluated in the emergency room setting. Although this option is not always well received by the person involved, it is the best and may be the only choice if someone is at risk for killing himself or herself.

Compliance
extent that behavior follows medical advice, such as by taking prescribed treatments.

Relapse
the return of symptoms of a mental illness for which one is currently receiving active treatment.

30. My father died 6 months ago. Since then, my mother refuses to leave the house, stating that she is still in mourning. What should I do?

Anthony's comment:

Everyone grieves at his or her own pace. Bereavement expands across all areas. This can even include the loss of a pet, which I recently experienced. I considered my pet my best friend after having her for 15 years in my life. After the loss, I did not want to celebrate holidays or spend time with friends. I have been grieving for six months and still have difficulty with the loss. Bereavement differs for all people and ultimately you have to grieve for the time that is right for yourself. I used to believe that the sooner you return to your normal activities, the better you are, but after I was diagnosed and treated with cancer, I realized you can not be expected to maintain a specific schedule. I had returned to my job too soon at that time, and it was a big mistake - the return to "normalcy" did not actually create the best conditions for my personal recovery, and ultimately created worse circumstances to deal with.

Bereavement can be a complicated process for many people and differs between cultural groups as well as between individuals. Symptoms of grief can look the same as symptoms of major depression. Death of a spouse is extremely stressful and often precipitates a major depressive episode. Defining the start point of such an episode in the context of bereavement can be difficult. Generally speaking, after an undefined period, a process toward moving on begins. Funerals and memorial services are ritual-based events that help provide a sense of closure for many people to help them recover from their grief. If there is no evidence of efforts toward this recovery, with poor functioning in work and/or relationships persisting, then the presence of a clinical depression is more likely. If suicidal thoughts occur, perhaps associated with wishes to be with the spouse again, depression that requires treatment is likely present. In such circumstances, it is best to seek professional help. It may be difficult to convince the grieving person to go for an evaluation, but helping set up the appointment, attending the appointment, and even insisting that consultation be sought can be useful. Again, if suicidal thinking is believed to be present, going to a local emergency room may be necessary if treatment interventions are refused.

31. My mother has been drinking wine daily since my father died. Could she be depressed?

One risk of untreated depression is the development of **co-morbid** substance abuse, including alcohol abuse. Alcohol and drugs make people feel better temporarily, but this effect is only temporary; as the high wears off, despair can set in. After the death of a spouse or other close family member, if excessive drinking develops, it

Co-morbid
the presence of two or more mental disorders, such as depression and anxiety.

is reasonable to presume that a depression is present. Alcohol abuse can often be missed in older women, particularly if it involves only consumption of wine or beer. Alcohol abuse can cause depression itself—in such circumstances, recovery from the substance abuse usually leads to resolution of the depression. Oftentimes, depression precipitates the abuse of alcohol and/or drugs and thus will need treatment to promote recovery from the substance abuse.

32. I have been treated for depression in the past. Can I prevent an episode in the future?

Anthony's comment:

I believe there are things you can do, such as relaxation activities of any kind, avoiding high stress situations, and engagement in physical activities.

Although many people who recover completely from a depressive episode never become depressed again, more than half of people who have been depressed will have another episode at some point in the future. The risk for future episodes increases with more episodes of depression. Although there are no specific preventive measures that can be taken, there are ways to lower the risk for recurrence, including reducing stress levels and developing problem-solving strategies. Exercise, good nutrition, and adequate sleep promote a healthy sense of wellness, which can ward off negative effects of stress. In addition, a lack of adequate sleep can be associated with increased irritability, malaise, and poor functioning during the day, which may precipitate depression in someone who is vulnerable. Some people find that the use of relaxation techniques such as meditation or yoga reduces stress levels. Psychotherapy helps an individual develop new coping styles and insights into his or her responses to negative events. With increased self-awareness and self-esteem, there is a reduced vulnerability to situations that could precipitate depression. Also, early recognition of the signs and symptoms of depression allows for early treatment intervention, which can hasten recovery.

33. My mother is depressed but refuses to see anyone. What can I do?

Anthony's comment:

My mother would not seek help for what I believed was depression. She drank excessive alcohol. It wasn't until my friend's mother took my mother to an Alcoholics Anonymous meeting, where my mother was listening to other people and their stories and became scared – that she then realized she should try to take care of herself. As a result she stopped her drinking with the help of her internist. While she never did seek mental health professional assistance, her internist was able to help her stop drinking and deal with her depression. You may have to be patient in waiting for your family member to get the help she needs and to acknowledge that there is a problem.

This can be a very complicated situation for the family members of a person who appears to be suffering from depression. Because of the stigma of mental illness, many depressed persons never seek treatment. This may be more likely based on age (older), gender (male), or ethnic and cultural identity (mental illness has a greater stigma in many cultures). An individual with close ties might want to encourage the affected person to seek treatment in any way possible. Perhaps the person will not see a psychiatrist but will agree to meet with a social worker. Suggest a consultation first, after which treatment can be considered. Maybe the person would be willing to speak with a clergy person at his or her place of worship. One could accompany the person to his or her next family doctor or internist appointment, where he or she might be willing to have you communicate concerns to the doctor. Making an initial appointment with a mental health practitioner on behalf of the affected individual may be enough to motivate him or her to seek help, especially if you agree to attend the appointment as well. If, however, a person absolutely refuses to meet with anyone, a decision needs to be made as to potential for dangerousness to self or others. For example, if suicidal ideation is suspected, local emergency personnel can be called to take the person to the emergency room. He or she may be angry with this, but if suicide is a possibility, the risk is worth taking. Some communities have mobile crisis units available in which a team of mental health practitioners comes to the home to evaluate the person in crisis. Information about home-based mental health services for persons in crisis can usually be obtained from the community or city hospitals that sponsor such programs.

34. My spouse is returning from active duty overseas. What is the risk for depression?

Depending on where your spouse is stationed, the risk for depression may be no higher than the general population, or it may be significantly increased because of his or her location and assigned duties. The closer your spouse is to combat, both geographically and occupationally, the higher the potential for developing posttraumatic stress disorder and resulting alcoholism and depression. Some recent evidence has shown that the highest rates of posttraumatic stress disorder and resulting depression come from soldiers who have fired on and witnessed their enemy being killed in contrast to being injured. A recent study on returning Iraqi soldiers, however, demonstrated that being fired on or ambushed did result in higher rates of posttraumatic stress disorder symptoms.

Nearly every soldier who returns from combat will suffer from some symptoms of trauma, although most will turn these experiences into constructive, character-building memories that will serve them well in their future endeavors. However, in those soldiers who continue to experience symptoms consistent with the diagnosis of posttraumatic stress disorder, the rates of depression approach 50%. The longer those symptoms persist, the more resistant to treatment they become; thus, it is important that they be treated as soon as possible. This is often the tricky part, as it is hard to get a spouse returning from combat to admit to having a problem, as he or she would feel that this admits to weakness and failure as a soldier (see Question 72 for further discussion on this topic).

PART FOUR

Treatment

What are the different types of treatment for depression?

Does the type of depression that I have determine the type of treatment I need?

What are the different types of talk therapies, and what do they do?

More ...

35. What are the different types of treatment for depression?

Types of treatment for depression fall into two broad categories: psychosocial and **pharmacological**. Within each category are many choices. Psychosocial treatments include individual therapies, group therapies, vocational services, family/couples therapies, as well as others. Furthermore, there are different types of individual therapies, such as supportive, insight oriented, or cognitive–behavioral. There are also various levels of treatment settings, ranging from private practice settings, outpatient clinic settings, day treatment or partial hospital programs, and inpatient treatment.

Pharmacological
pertaining to all chemicals that, when ingested, cause a physiological process to occur in the body.

Pharmacologic treatment involves the use of medications from various groups, such as antidepressants, **anticonvulsants**, **antipsychotics**, or **anxiolytics**. Psychotropics are those medicines that are primarily used in psychiatric care for the treatment of mental disorders, including depression. However, there is often a crossover use of medicines from other medical specialties, such as from neurology, wherein antiseizure medications (anticonvulsants) are frequently found to have **efficacy** in the treatment of many psychiatric conditions.

Anticonvulsant
a drug that controls or prevents seizures.

Antipsychotic
a drug that treats psychotic symptoms, such as hallucinations, delusions, and thought disorders.

Anxiolytic
a substance that relieves subjective and objective symptoms of anxiety.

Efficacy
the capacity to produce a desired effect.

As part of an evaluation, your clinician will consider the most appropriate treatment plan for your depression. For a mild depression, psychotherapy alone may be recommended first. For more severe depressions, both medication and therapy may be recommended. If already in psychotherapy, your therapist may refer you to a psychiatrist for a medication evaluation if there are concerns about the level of response, the severity of

Table 3

Therapy	Duration	Illness/Focus	Theory
Psychoanalytic or psychodynamic	few months to few years	personality disorders, coping skills	unconscious conflicts from childhood
Behavioral	6-20 sessions	anxiety disorders, depression, psychosomatic symptoms	symptom reinforcement
Cognitive	10-20 sessions	depression, obsessive-compulsive disorder	negative thoughts
Interpersonal	12 sessions	depression	relationship focused
Dialectical behavioral	one year or greater	borderline personality disorder	reduction of self-injurious behaviors
Psycho-educational	long-term	families of schizophrenic patients	support and education
Supportive	brief	acute grief reactions	reinforcing patient's strengths
Group	open-ended or time-limited	mood disorders, anxiety disorders, schizophrenia	support and education
Family	short to long-term	family roles, support, education, dynamics	various

symptoms, or confounding co-morbid conditions. The type of therapy chosen can depend on many factors such as cost, duration, or patient fit (Table 3). Frequency of psychotherapy typically starts at once per week but may be more or less often depending on your individual needs or therapy type.

As part of the treatment plan, the treatment setting also needs to be determined. Most individuals can be treated in private office settings or outpatient clinic settings. Sometimes, a higher level of structure is needed in which more services can be provided, on a daily basis, such as in a day treatment program. If impairments are severe or if safety is in question, hospitalization may be warranted. Within the hospital, several modalities of treatment are provided on a daily basis, making the treatment more intense.

36. Does the type of depression that I have determine the type of treatment I need?

Treatments for depression work for all types, and typically, the specific type of depression does not change the treatment approach drastically. It does, however, inform as to certain patterns of response to treatments, as well as to the degree of intervention that may be necessary. For example, an individual with major depression with psychotic features is more apt to require hospitalization than an individual with dysthymic disorder. Some subtypes of depression have evidence of better response to certain treatments. For example, an atypical depression has classically been considered more responsive to a specific medication class, called the MAOIs. Depression with melancholic features may respond better to tricyclic antidepressants (TCAs). Seasonal depression responds best to a treatment called light therapy. The presence of bipolar disorder usually means that a mood stabilizer will be a necessary part of the treatment, as the use of an antidepressant without a mood stabilizer in a bipolar individual puts the person at risk for the development of a manic episode.

37. What are the different types of talk therapies, and what do they do?

Once you receive a consultation, the clinician will make recommendations as to the most appropriate treatment or therapeutic approach for your circumstances. He or she may be able to use that approach or can refer you to persons who specialize in a specific approach. Many therapists use a combination of therapeutic approaches in their work. Some of the different approaches are as follows.

Psychodynamic therapy assumes the depression is due to unresolved, unconscious conflicts from childhood. It is based on the classic psychoanalytic approach that Sigmund Freud developed. The therapist uses the concepts of **transference**, **countertransference**, **resistance**, free association, and dreams in order to help the patient develop insight into patterns in relationships that can then effect change. It is a nondirective therapy. Although classic analytical therapy can last for years, with sessions 4 to 5 days per week, psychodynamic therapy may be shorter in duration, with sessions 1 to 3 times per week. Controlled research studies examining the efficacy of this type of therapy are minimal because of the nature of this type of therapy. It is often a helpful treatment approach for those with chronic coping difficulties or with personality disorders.

Transference

the unconscious assignment of feelings and attitudes to a therapist from previous important relationships in one's life (parents and siblings).

Countertransferance

the attitudes, opinions, and behaviors that a therapist attributes to his or her patient, not based on the true nature of the patient but rather the biased nature of the therapist.

Resistance

the tendency to avoid treatment interventions, often unconsciously (e.g., missed appointments, arriving late, forgetting medication).

Interpersonal therapy conceptualizes depression in a patient with the three components of symptom formation, social functioning, and personality factors. It focuses on the patient's social, or interpersonal, functioning, with expected improvement in symptoms. The

Interpersonal therapy

a form of therapy that focuses strictly on current relationships and conflicts within them.

goal is to improve communication skills and self-esteem. It is a brief and highly structured, manual-based psychotherapy. Areas of social functioning that may be addressed are interpersonal disputes, role transitions, grief, and interpersonal deficits. Therapy is focused and brief in duration, typically lasting 12 to 16 sessions. Research studies have shown it to be an effective treatment for depression.

Cognitive–behavioral therapy
an approach in psychotherapy, during which the therapist focuses on a self-defeating quality in order to replace it with a more positive thought and behavior.

Cognitive–behavioral therapy assumes the depression is due to a pattern of negative thinking. It works to help patients identify and change inaccurate perceptions of themselves and situations. It also is brief in duration and manually based, typically lasting for 10 to 20 sessions. It typically involves the use of homework assignments between sessions. Research studies have shown it to be an effective treatment for depression and some anxiety disorders (see Question 39 for further discussion on cognitive–behavioral therapy).

38. How do I choose a therapist and a therapy approach?

Choosing a therapist can be an overwhelming task. One look in the yellow pages shows lists of names, and not everyone lists in the yellow pages. One factor to consider is that there are many possible credentials of therapists. Some people identify themselves as therapists but do not have credentials that require licensure within their state. In general, a licensed practitioner will have been through a screening process that usually involves testing within their field. The level of training is another consideration. There are master's levels (social workers), doctorate levels (psychologists), as well as medical doctorate levels (psychiatrists) who conduct psychotherapy. Clinicians of various credentials may then have further training within a specific area of psychotherapy, such as psychoanalysis.

If you think that you will need medication, it may be more fruitful to see a psychiatrist who also performs psychotherapy. Because of cost considerations, however, this option is not always feasible. Many insurance plans will provide reimbursement for a master's level therapist only, and fees are usually less than that for psychologists or psychiatrists. If there is a specific treatment modality in mind, one method of finding a therapist is to obtain referrals from professional societies for that specific modality. If modality is not the issue of concern, referrals can be obtained from a primary care physician. Questions may be asked of the therapist over the phone and a consultation arranged. If you are uncomfortable with the therapist after the consultation, it is important to consider the reasons for your discomfort. Sometimes individual psychological issues are **projected** onto the therapist immediately and thus are avoided by failing to continue to see the therapist. However, a fit with the therapist's style needs to be achieved in order to develop a working relationship.

39. What is cognitive–behavioral therapy?

Cognitive–behavioral therapy is based on two separate theoretical models, both cognitive and behavioral. Cognitive models are based on the premise that cognitions, or thoughts, determine emotions and behavior. **Automatic thoughts** are one type of cognition that may be distorted by errors of thinking such as **overgeneralization**, **catastrophic thinking**, jumping to

Projected
the attribution of one's own unconscious thoughts and feelings to others.

Automatic thoughts
thoughts that occur spontaneously whenever a specific, common event occurs in one's life and that are often associated with depression.

Overgeneralization
the act of taking a specific event and applying one's reactions to that event to an array of events that are not really in the same class but are perceived as such.

Catastrophic thinking
a type of automatic thought during which the individual quickly assumes the worst outcome for a given situation.

conclusions, or personalization. Errors in thinking tend to be more frequent and intense in depression as well as in other psychiatric disorders. Behavioral models are based on theories of learning such as by modeling or by reinforcement to certain responses.

Cognitive–behavioral therapy is an approach that uses techniques based on the models described previously here. A greater emphasis on cognitive approaches or on behavioral approaches may be taken depending on the disorder and the stage of treatment. Cognitive techniques include

- Psychoeducation
- Modifying automatic thoughts
- Modifying **schemas**

Behavioral techniques include

- Activity scheduling
- Breathing control
- **Contingency contracting**
- Desensitization/relaxation training
- Exposure and **flooding**
- Social skills training
- **Thought stopping**/distraction

Through many of these techniques, patients learn to manage their anxiety and reactions to stress appropriately. Exposure training is a technique that uses **graded exposure** to a high-anxiety situation by breaking the task into small steps that are focused on one by one.

Cognitive–behavioral therapy has been the best studied form of psychotherapy and has been shown to treat

Schema
representations in the mind of the world that affect perception of and response to the environment.

Contingency contracting
use of reinforcers, or rewards to modify behaviors.

Flooding
exposure to the maximal level of anxiety as quickly as possible.

Thought stopping
a technique used to suppress repetitive thoughts.

Graded exposure
gradual exposure to situations ranging from least to most anxiety-provoking.

depression effectively. It is probably more appropriate in cases of mild to moderate depression that is acute. Treatment typically lasts 3 to 6 months with 10 to 20 weekly sessions. The patient is expected to be an active participant in trying new strategies and will be expected to do homework.

40. Are there any risks from engaging in psychotherapy?

Psychotherapy appears, on the surface, to be one of the most benign forms of medical therapies. There is (usually) no physical contact. No medications are prescribed. Only words are exchanged between people—nothing more. However, never underestimate the power of words. There is a parable that may be recalled from childhood: "Sticks and stones may break my bones but names will never hurt me." Such a parable was created to provide comfort from the emotional wounds received from being called names. One would not need to recite such a parable if words did not hurt! Words carry power. Just as psychotherapy has the power to heal, it also has the power to harm. The harms vary from lack of progress to outright abuse. Most harm from psychotherapy comes from what are known as boundary violations between the therapist and the patient. The most obvious boundary violation stems from sexual or physical relationships that can develop between the therapist and patient. In many states, this boundary violation is considered a criminal offense because the power differential between the patient and therapist is so great as to put the patient in a particularly vulnerable position.

Other boundary violations are not as obvious. Simple exchanges of personal information between the patient and therapist are often considered to be boundary violations and may or may not lead to more serious offenses on the part of the therapist. The potential dangers are that they may lead to friendly meetings that move beyond the office, and friendly meetings may turn more intimate. Although many patients may experience their therapists as friends, such feelings generated are known in therapy as transference. Transference is an artificial relationship that the patient projects onto the therapist. In **insight-oriented** or **dynamic** (Freudian) psychotherapy, a transference relationship is intentionally created to allow the therapist to understand a patient's outside relationships better. This in turn allows the therapist to help a patient develop insight or greater understanding into the unconscious motives behind his or her relationships so that healthy interactions can be learned.

Insight-oriented
a form of psychotherapy that focuses on one's developmental history and interpersonal relationships.

Dynamic
referring to a type of therapy that focuses on one's interpersonal relationships, developmental experiences, and the transference relationship with his or her therapist.

Therapists also develop transference relationships to their patients known as countertransference. If the therapist is unaware of his or her countertransference, behavior toward patients reflects the therapist's own outside relationships. If such relationships are problematic, a patient may be made to feel that he or she is experiencing problems that are really the problems of the therapist. Patients often idolize their therapist, which makes patients particularly vulnerable to the influence of their therapist's words.

A notable example of the vulnerability patients can have in therapy occurred a few years ago when some cases were made public of patients believing through their therapists' suggestions that their parents sexually abused them. The process by which this occurred came about through the implantation of false memories on the part of their therapists. The therapists did not do this intentionally. However, in their zeal to associate certain symptoms that their patients presented with to a history of sexual abuse, they began to gradually convince their patients that they had repressed memories of abuse. Once they had convinced their patients of past abuse, false memories could easily be constructed by asking them to imagine being abused or by implanting false memories through hypnosis. "False memory syndrome" was coined, and several high-profile legal cases occurred in which patients sued their therapists for psychological damages as a result of the patients taking legal action against their parents based on their false memories.

How can one avoid such risks? One must rely primarily on referrals and word of mouth from friends as well as other professionals. Generally, one's primary care doctor has developed relationships with various therapists over the years and knows their work. Success in therapy is not dependent on the academic degree of the therapist as much as it is on the therapist's training and experience in treating patients. Secondarily, one needs to maintain an open mind to make changes if uncomfortable with a particular therapist, no matter how skilled he or she may be. Chemistry between patient and therapist is needed, and no amount of training provides that for any particular patient. Success in therapy depends on how one feels about the therapy sessions as well as the motivation from the therapist to "do the work" outside of therapy in order to make the changes needed.

41. How does psychotherapy work if depression is due to a chemical imbalance?

Anthony's comment:

Psychotherapy is a broad area of treatment with different modalities available. My experience with psychotherapy is that is gives you the insight to allow yourself to make better choices. It is my opinion that psychotherapy has been a necessary part of my treatment, as it has made me able to look inward to figure out why I engage in certain behaviors. Once you have some degree of insight you can ease your situation by avoiding certain behaviors. Psychotherapy was of use to me as a long-term treatment over a few years. While I no longer continue with regular sessions, I still choose to have periodic contact via phone or face-to-face sessions.

Every thought, feeling, and behavior is associated with a chemical change in the brain. If thoughts, feelings, and behaviors occur with a repeated pattern, structural changes can occur in the brain as well. Learning and memory involve complex chemical changes that lead to permanent structural changes in brain anatomy. For example, consider the first time that one learns how to drive a car. It requires conscious processing of complex pieces of information and integrating the information into an organized behavioral pattern. The powers of concentration at that time could be exhausting. However, with practice, the skill becomes second nature as the brain adapts the skill so that much of it occurs unconsciously. Over-learned behavior such as that ultimately leads to structural and biochemical changes in the brain.

The chemistry and structure of the brain can change via one of three methods: (1) change in the environment, (2) change in brain chemistry via chemical modification with the use of psychotropic medication, and (3) learning how to modify the environment or perception of the environment by developing new skills.

Moving, changing jobs, and getting married or divorced are examples of the first method, whereas psychopharmacology is the second. Psychotherapy is the third method. Brain-imaging studies have repeatedly demonstrated, for example, that changes occur in the same brain regions of patients with obsessive–compulsive disorder on fluoxetine as those receiving **cognitive–behavioral therapy**. Each of these methods has its own inherent costs and benefits, and therefore, none can be considered inherently better or worse than another. The effects of all three methods are generally cumulative; thus, in order for one to have the best chance of recovery from depression, a combination of two to three methods is generally warranted.

Cognitive–behavioral therapy

a combination of cognitive and behavioral approaches in psychotherapy, during which the therapist focuses on automatic thoughts and behavior of a self-defeating quality in order to make one more conscious of them and replace them with more positive thoughts and behaviors.

42. What are the different types of medication used to treat depression? How does my doctor choose a medicine?

Medication choices include many medications within the following classes:

- Tricyclic antidepressants (TCAs)
- Monoamine oxidase inhibitors (MAOIs)
- Selective serotonin reuptake inhibitors (SSRIs)
- Others

TCAs and MAOIs are the oldest antidepressants. They are effective treatments but have many problematic side effects. In addition, they can be unsafe to use

Table 4 Dietary restrictions while taking an MAOI*

Matured or aged cheeses
Fermented or dried meats
Fava and broad bean pods
Tap beers
Marmite yeast extract
Sauerkraut
Soy sauce and other soy products
Smoked, pickled, or fermented fish
Improperly stored meats, fish, and dairy products

*This list is intended to be a general guideline only; more specific information on restrictions as well as permissible foods should be obtained from your doctor

in patients with certain medical conditions and in older persons. MAOIs require strict adherence to a dietary plan that is free of tyramine (Table 4). Although these medications are effective for treatment of depression, they are now typically reserved for use after a person's symptoms have not improved on one of the newer medications available. The most commonly prescribed TCAs are desipramine and nortriptyline because of their better tolerated side effect profiles (see Table 5 for a list of available TCAs and MAOIs).

The first SSRI to enter the market was fluoxetine (Prozac) in the late 1980s. Because of its low side-effect profile relative to the TCAs and MAOIs, fluoxetine quickly became the most popular antidepressant. Several SSRIs have come on the market since (Table 6). Because SSRIs as a group are the most commonly prescribed antidepressants, the decision as to choice of medication is often in deciding between the SSRIs available. There is no good evidence that any SSRI is better than another in the treatment of depression or any of the anxiety disorders. The choice of SSRI has more to do with side-effect profiles and potential for drug–drug interactions. **Discontinuation**

Table 5 Tricyclic Antidepressants and Monoamine Oxidase Inhibitors

TCAs
clomipramine (Anafranil)
amitriptyline (Elavil)
doxepin (Sinequan)
trimipramine (Surmontil)
amoxapine (Asendin)
protriptyline (Vivactil)
desipramine (Norpramin)
nortriptyline (Pamelor, Aventyl)
imipramine (Tofranil)
maprotiline (Ludiomil)
MAOIs
phenelzine (Nardil)
tranylcypromine (Parnate)

Table 6 Selective Serotonin Reuptake Inhibitors

fluoxetine (Prozac)
sertraline (Zoloft)
paroxetine (Paxil)
fluvoxamine (Luvox)
citalopram (Celexa)
escitalopram (Lexapro)

syndromes are least likely from fluoxetine and are more likely from paroxetine. Fluoxetine may be a better choice for someone who tends to miss doses of medication. On the other hand, because of its long **half-life**, adverse effects will take longer to dissipate after discontinuation of the drug. In terms of potential interactions with other medications, fluoxetine, paroxetine, and fluvoxamine have the highest potential for such interactions. Sertraline, citalopram, and escitalopram have a lower risk for interactions. Cost may be a

Discontinuation syndrome
physical symptoms that occur when a drug is suddenly stopped.

Half-life
the time it takes for half of the blood concentration of a medication to be eliminated from the body.

factor in medication choice as well, with fluoxetine and paroxetine being available in generic forms.

Medications classified under "other" have various mechanisms of action (see Table 7). Bupropion blocks the reuptake of dopamine and norepinephrine. Bupropion does not have significant drug–drug interactions and is not associated with sexual dysfunction. Venlafaxine and duloxetine are dual reuptake inhibitors of both norepinephrine and serotonin (and to a lesser extent, dopamine). They have similar side effect profiles to the SSRIs but have the advantage of working through two neurotransmitter systems. Mirtazapine causes increased levels of serotonin and norepinephrine by blocking the inhibition of their release (both serotonin and norepinephrine act to turn off their own release by interacting with receptors on the sending neuron). Trazodone and nefazodone are chemically similar (trazodone is an older antidepressant), blocking serotonin reuptake as well as blocking some types of serotonin receptors directly. Trazodone is very sedating and is mainly used for insomnia, and nefazodone is not

Table 7 Antidepressants with Other Mechanisms of Action

Name	Mechanism of Action
venlafaxine (Effexor)	serotonin and norepinephrine reuptake inhibition
duloxetine (Cymbalta)	serotonin and norepinephrine reuptake inhibition
mirtazapine (Remeron)	blocks the inhibition of serotonin and norepinephrine release
trazodone (Desyrel)	serotonin receptor blockade and reuptake inhibition
nefazodone (Serzone)	serotonin receptor blockade and reuptake inhibition
bupropion (Wellbutrin)	norepinephrine and dopamine reuptake inhibition

first-line because of its association with some cases of liver failure.

Typically, the first decision regarding antidepressant choice is between the newer classes. All antidepressants are effective for depression, but the choice of type will likely depend on side-effect profiles, patient characteristics, physician preference, and cost. Some insurance plans have formularies restricting use to a specific medication. In these circumstances, the physician would need to explain the rationale for choosing a nonformulary medicine over a formulary one. Side-effect profiles for the different medication classes noted previously here are listed in Table 8. Appendix B lists all antidepressants with their dosing ranges, formulations, and approximate cost per month.

In addition to antidepressants, many other medications are used in the treatment of depression: anticonvulsants, antipsychotics, and **benzodiazepines**. Typically, these medications are used to address specific co-morbid conditions or symptoms that are not addressed by the antidepressant. In cases of partial response to an antidepressant, there may be medications prescribed for **augmentation**, including buspirone, thyroid hormone, or even a stimulant such as methylphenidate.

Benzodiazepine
a drug that is part of a class of medication with sedative and anxiolytic effects.

Augmentation
in pharmacotherapy, a strategy of using a second medication to enhance the positive effects of an existing medication in the regimen.

43. What are the side effects of medication for depression?

Anthony's comment:

There are many side effects from medication. It is best to be informed of these in advance. When I took Lexapro, I felt that some of my senses were numbed. My libido was gone too. It returned however when I went off the medication. I spoke with my doctor about it. Now I take Wellbutrin on which I

Table 8 Adverse Effects of Antidepressants by Class*

Medication class	Potential Adverse Effects
SSRIs	nausea, diarrhea, insomnia, anxiety, nervousness, dizziness, somnolence, tremor, decreased libido, sweating, anorexia, dry mouth, headache, sexual dysfunction, serotonin syndrome
TCAs	dry mouth, constipation, nausea, anorexia, weight gain, sweating, increased appetite, nervousness, decreased libido, dizziness, tremor, somnolence, blurred vision, tachycardia, urinary hesitancy, hypotension, cardiac toxicity
MAOIs	dizziness, headache, drowsiness, hypotension, insomnia, agitation, dry mouth, constipation, nausea, urinary hesitancy, weight gain, edema, sexual dysfunction, increased liver enzymes, toxic food and drug interactions
Others (drugs listed separately)	
bupropion (Wellbutrin)	weight loss, dry mouth, rash, sweating, agitation, dizziness, insomnia, nausea, abdominal pain, weakness, headache, blurred vision, constipation, tremor, rapid heart rate, ringing in ears, seizures
venlafaxine (Effexor)	sweating, nausea, constipation, decreased appetite, vomiting, insomnia, somnolence, dry mouth, dizziness, nervousness, tremor, blurred vision, sexual dysfunction, rapid heart rate, hypertension
duloxetine (Cymbalta)	nausea, dry mouth, constipation, loss of appetite, fatigue, drowsiness, dizziness, sweating, blurred vision, rash, itching, sexual dysfunction, tremor, unusual bleeding
mirtazopine (Remeron)	somnolence, appetite increase, weight gain, dizziness, dry mouth, constipation, hypotension, abnormal dreams, flu syndrome, low blood cell counts
nefazodone (Serzone)	somnolence, dry mouth, nausea, dizziness, insomnia, agitation, constipation, abnormal vision, confusion, liver failure
trazodone (Desyrel)	sedation, hypotension, dizziness, blurred vision, headache, loss of appetite, sweating, restlessness, rapid heart rate, prolonged erection

*Listed adverse effects are not exhaustive of side effects as reported in the Physicians' Desk Reference. Rather more common effects within each group were included, as well as some more serious effects. Side effect profiles of medications within a class may vary. Any concern about an adverse effect from a medication should be discussed with your doctor.

feel much better. While antidepressants can numb your senses and make you sluggish, the body usually adjusts. It is important to discuss side effects with your doctor because there may be solutions or alternatives. When I was unhappy with side effects, I stopped the medication, but that wasn't the best thing to do, because then I began to relapse with my depression.

Side effects can occur with all medications, not just psychotropic medications. In depression, however, medications are taken for long periods, and thus, some side effects may not be tolerable because of the duration of treatment required. Side effects vary both within a class of medications and between classes. Typically, one class of medications shares similar side effects; however, if one medicine within a class causes a specific side effect (e.g., nausea), it is not necessarily the case that another medicine within the same class will cause the same side effect.

Table 8 lists some of the more common side effects from specific medication classes. Some medications have rare but potentially serious side effects (Table 9).

Table 9 Potentially Serious Side Effects of Antidepressants

SSRIs	serotonin syndrome
TCAs	cardiac arrhythmia
MAOIs	malignant hypertension
bupropion	seizure
trazodone	prolonged erection (priapism)
nefazodone	liver failure
venlafaxine	hyponatremia, bleeding, hypertension
duloxetine	low blood cell counts
mirtazapine	low blood cell counts

all antidepressants now have warnings for possible suicidal behavior in children and adolescents.

Your doctor should go over these with you. Some side effects can be useful in certain situations. For example, in a person who has insomnia, a more sedating antidepressant may be helpful when taken in the evening. In someone with a poor appetite, a medication with an associated increase in appetite may be desired.

Rather than discontinuing a medication when there is a suspected, bothersome side effect, it is important to speak with your doctor first. Some side effects are transient or can be easily alleviated by another remedy (e.g., ibuprofen for headache). Stopping medications abruptly when any side effect occurs may cause a discontinuation syndrome, as well as may prematurely interrupt a potentially helpful treatment intervention. If possible, it is best to remain on a treatment for at least a few days, as some perceived side effects could be associated with unrelated conditions (e.g., viral infection). Bear in mind that scientific studies that compare an active medication to a **placebo** (sugar pill) have reported "side effects" in the placebo group as well. If a suspected effect seems dangerous for any reason, it certainly is most prudent to stop the medication until you are able to speak with a doctor and if necessary receive an evaluation in an emergency setting.

Placebo

an inert substance that when ingested causes absolutely no physiological process to occur but may have psychological effects.

44. Will I become addicted to the medication?

The one major concern for many patients who take these medications for years is the fear that they are addicted to the medication. **Addiction** is a complicated and controversial issue that bears some explaining. From a medical standpoint, addiction is defined as

Addiction

continued use of a mood-altering substance despite physical, psychological, or social harm.

pursuit of a substance in such a manner that the pursuit and use of it consumes so much time and energy for the person to the exclusion of the majority of, if not all of, important activities in that person's life. Therefore, anything that gives pleasure causing one to pursue it with abandon is potentially addictive—from gambling to sex to drugs and all variations on those themes. By that simple definition, no antidepressant has proven to be addictive, and very few psychiatric medications have shown to be addictive as well. Many people do, however, become dependent on various prescription medications, and this is where confusion reigns. Dependency is defined medically by the fact that physiologically measurable changes occur in the body after repeated administration of a drug. The most obvious drug that people think about in terms of dependency includes most of the prescription pain medications that are called opiates. Everyone who takes these medications on a regular basis will become dependent on them. The confusion between dependency and addiction stems from the fact that with dependency comes withdrawal when the drug is removed abruptly from the body, which can lead to craving for the drug. Because a drug like an opiate can make one high, is often pursued with abandon, and does cause dependency, people often mistake dependency for addiction.

Dependency and addiction may or may not be linked depending on the drug. For example, most anticonvulsant medications, many antihypertensive medications, and all steroid medications cause dependency, but no one would ever consider these drugs addictive. In stark contrast, many hallucinogens and stimulants do not cause any measurable physiologic changes in the body that one could absolutely label dependency, and nevertheless, these are some of the most highly addictive substances known to humans. Where do antidepressants and other psychiatric medications fit on this continuum? Most antidepressants cause some level of physiologic dependency, especially the TCAs. Some mood stabilizers and antipsychotic medications (particularly the older ones) also cause some physiologic dependency. Any drug, whether prescription medication or street drug, that causes dependency, must be tapered over time, or one risks developing withdrawal.

Three types of discontinuation syndromes can occur when you stop a medication that you have been taking regularly for a significant period of time: withdrawal, rebound, and recurrence. Withdrawal occurs when a drug or medication is abruptly stopped. It is accompanied by clear physiologically measurable changes, including vital sign changes, skin color and temperature changes, and psychological distress. For some drugs, such as benzodiazepines, this can be a life-threatening emergency. For this reason, one needs to always consult a physician when deciding to discontinue a medication to see whether such a withdrawal could occur. Rebound occurs when the symptoms for which one was receiving the medication become transiently worse than the symptoms one had before treatment. This is a potential risk for any sleep medication from which rebound insomnia can be very severe. However, this is a transient effect and abates within days. Unfortunately, most people do not realize that rebound is expected and transient, and they immediately go back on their sleeping medications. Rebound generally is not accompanied by any physiologic changes. Recurrence is simply the return of symptoms for which one originally received the medication. Recurrence is more delayed in the time line after stopping a medication than either withdrawal or rebound. Typically, if one begins to experience symptoms as early as a few days after stopping antidepressant medications, this actually represents rebound or minor withdrawal (no measurable physiologic changes) that is commonly known as a discontinuation syndrome. Rarely are the symptoms caused by recurrence. It is generally a good idea to taper the medications. When the medications are appropriately tapered, any symptoms that return can properly be attributed to recurrence, and thus, increasing the medication back to a therapeutic dose may be a wise choice. In summary, clearly, although these medications can cause various discontinuation syndromes, they are *not* addictive.

45. Will I gain weight from the medication?

Anne's comment:

One of the difficulties in experiencing weight gain caused by medication is the desire for the patient to stop taking what has been prescribed. In treating my adolescent daughter for bipolar disorder, weight gain has been a critical issue. Her doctor has been very sensitive to her feelings about her weight and willing to try different medications when one or another caused significant weight gain. As a result of the doctor's sensitivity, my daughter did not take the risk of discontinuing her medication. It was also important for her that family members did not make critical remarks while her weight fluctuated during the course of trying to find the right balance of medication.

Potential weight gain is a very real concern for many patients. The answer to this question is not so straightforward. As a group, the older antidepressants have been classically associated with weight gain (tricyclics, MAOIs). When the SSRIs first entered the market, they were believed to have no associated weight gain as a group, and some even were found to cause weight loss (e.g., Prozac). If the side-effect profiles are looked up in the *Physicians' Desk Reference*, weight gain is not noted for most of the SSRIs. Keep in mind that side-effect profiles are typically developed from the early studies of medications, which are conducted over the short term (i.e., several weeks). In the short term, for example, fluoxetine use can result in weight loss. In clinical practice, however, many physicians have found that SSRIs can be associated with weight gain over the long term. Although clinical trials have typically found that weight gain does not differ significantly from placebo, uncontrolled studies have noted weight gain over the long term. Paroxetine appears to be more associated with weight gain clinically than the other SSRIs. Citalopram has been reported to have early weight gain. There may be an increase in carbohydrate craving associated with SSRIs as a possible mechanism.

It is certainly plausible that weight gain over the long term may be independent of SSRI use in some people. Obesity has become an epidemic in this country regardless of medication use. More long-term controlled studies are needed to compare weight gain over time between antidepressant users and those who are not. Keeping in mind the potential for weight gain, good nutrition and exercise should be part of the treatment.

Although data are not conclusive regarding weight gain with SSRIs, there are data supporting weight gain potential from the anticonvulsants that are prescribed for bipolar conditions and mood instability in general. Also, **atypical antipsychotics** and benzodiazepines as classes of medications are associated with weight gain as well.

Atypical antipsychotic
a second-generation antipsychotic that has fewer neurologic side effects and also has mood-stabilizing effects.

When deciding what medication to use in treatment of depression, discussions about side effects should be undertaken with your doctor. The risk for weight gain needs to be balanced against the risk for untreated depression. Bupropion is one antidepressant that does not have weight gain associated with it and can be considered as one treatment option. Nefazodone also does not have weight gain associated with it, but because of recent concerns about liver toxicity, it is no longer a first-line treatment for depression.

46. How long will I have to stay on medication?

Anne's comment:

Medication has provided my spouse with the capacity to function at his highest level. He has been able to work for over 20 years without having to take a medical leave and to lead a full life, including time with family and friends. He remains in therapy, and his medications are adjusted as needed. For us, it is not a question of whether he should remain on medication. Like a diabetic who needs to monitor blood sugar levels and adjust insulin doses to feel well and take an active role in life, a person who suffers from chronic depression can remain well with appropriate and consistent treatment.

It is important to understand that antidepressant therapy is used for treatment of the acute illness as well as to maintain remission of the depression. Remission may be partial or full and can occur within 4 to 6 weeks after the initiation of medication. Full remission has occurred when there are no longer any symptoms. This is not, however, a good time to stop the medication. Many people stop their antidepressant treatment prematurely because they feel better. It may be thought that the medication is not needed anymore or even questioned whether the medication had anything to do at all with the improvement (particularly if there were no side effects). Close monitoring by your doctor can help to address questions of efficacy as well as to provide the feedback as to level of improvement. When medication is discontinued prematurely, a relapse or recurrence is likely to occur soon thereafter. A relapse occurs if there is a return of depression within the period of time known as remission, which is within 6 months of remission of symptoms. Recurrence occurs if depression returns during the period of recovery, which is after 6 months of remission. Statistically speaking, after remission of a depressive episode, there is highest risk for recurrence within the first year. The standard recommendation therefore is to continue antidepressant therapy for 9 months to 1 year after complete remission of symptoms. After one episode of depression, the risk for recurrence after a year in remission is similar to the baseline risk for depression. The more episodes of depression that occur over time, however, the higher is the risk for future episodes. In fact, a history of three or more episodes places patients at a greater than 80% risk for recurrence. Therefore, after two or more episodes (depending on severity), your doctor may recommend indefinite treatment with an antidepressant in order to reduce your risk for recurrence.

47. Is medication or therapy more effective for depression?

Anthony's comment:

Therapy is the first tool in treatment. Without self-awareness any further attempts at treatment are going to be difficult if not futile. If a medical professional deems it necessary medication can help one to cope better with depression. Neither medication nor therapy is particularly more effective than the other; for me personally it had to be both and I wouldn't have accepted any medicine unless there was the opportunity for discussion on my life circumstances.

Both medication and therapy are effective treatments for depression. The treatment choice depends on the severity of the episode. Mild depression is often effectively treated with cognitive–behavioral therapy or interpersonal therapy alone, for example. More severe forms of depression typically require the adjunctive use of medication. Some individuals only take medication, but studies have shown that the combination of medication with therapy can be the most effective. When taking medication, it is usually best to have some form of therapy at some point during the treatment in order to address the precipitating stressors. This would help develop coping mechanisms and problem-solving abilities and reduces the risk of recurrence under stressful circumstances in the future.

The most important factor in determining a positive outcome from either modality is that both forms of treatment require *commitment* to the treatment in order for it to work. Therapy requires regular attendance to appointments, communication with the therapist during the session, and for some forms of therapy, work on assignments between sessions. The process of therapy is not easy. It can be anxiety provoking, and one does not necessarily feel relief after each individual session. Relief comes over time with hard work on the issues. It may feel easier to cancel sessions or to terminate treatment prematurely, but then the therapy is not given a chance to be effective.

As for medication, its use requires daily compliance and regular communication with your doctor. It is often difficult for many people to remember to take a medication daily, twice a day, or more. Doses may be skipped. Missing doses regularly results in reduced efficacy of the medication. Sometimes a medication does not work right away. It becomes frustrating, and the medication treatment is abandoned prematurely. Oftentimes, when a person has a list of "ineffective" medication, many of them did not get adequate trials.

You may wish to try therapy alone first, and depending on progress, consider use of medication later. This route may be appropriate for milder cases of depression. Again, the more severe the depression, the more likely medication will also be necessary, as improvement in symptoms usually occurs more quickly with medication. Persistent, unremitting depression can be harmful because of its adverse physical and emotional effects as well as its associated risk for suicide. Therefore, the decision to initiate or hold off on medication needs to be made very carefully. Again, it is optimal to be in therapy while on medication, as the therapy will provide the skills needed to manage stressful situations in the future and will hopefully deter future depressive episodes.

48. My doctor thinks that I should have electroconvulsive therapy. I thought that was no longer used. What is it and what does it do?

Many myths exist surrounding the use of electroconvulsive therapy (**ECT**), which is a procedure that induces a seizure in the brain through an application of an electric current through the scalp. Although ECT is not a first-line treatment (and is typically only offered after several failed medication trials/repeated hospitalizations), it is a very effective treatment. It is very safe and is not painful. The patient is given anesthesia and a muscle relaxant for the procedure. For some patients, ECT is safer than medications, particularly for those with serious medical conditions for whom medication can be contraindicated and for pregnant woman who may not want to expose the fetus to a certain medication (e.g., lithium). ECT is growing in use in older depressed patients because of higher rates of concurrent medical illness and risks of toxicity from medication. Psychotic depressions are often refractory to medication, and thus, ECT may be considered early on in the treatment to avoid a prolonged course of medication trials.

ECT
electroconvulsive or shock therapy.

The risk of serious complication from ECT is 1 in 1,000. Cardiac complications are the most common adverse effects, which is why a pre-ECT evaluation includes evaluation of the cardiac system. Most potential cardiovascular complications can be avoided with the use of appropriate medications. Confusion and/or memory loss are also often common. Confusion is usually transient. Memory deficits may be for events before or after the procedure. Memory deficits usually resolve over weeks to months after, although occasionally there are more persistent memory difficulties.

Although ECT provides rapid improvement in symptoms of depression, there is a high rate of relapse—up to 50% within 6 months—and thus, either continuation/maintenance ECT or medication is recommended after the treatment course. Continuation ECT is usually provided only if continuation medication has not successfully prevented relapse or recurrence of depression in the past.

ECT is usually done in a hospital setting as an inpatient (outpatient ECT may be provided for maintenance ECT). Medications are typically tapered and discontinued before the treatment, and this process may need to occur in a hospital setting because of the risk for worsening depression and/or suicidality. ECT providers have received specialized training and certification. Although protocols may vary from state to state, usually more than one physician needs to evaluate the patient and determine that ECT is clinically appropriate.

Unfortunately, because of the media's negative portrayal of ECT over the years, even with the safety features in place, this very effective procedure is highly stigmatized and even illegal in some jurisdictions.

49. Are there any natural remedies for depression?

Alternative treatment

a treatment for a medical condition that has not undergone scientific studies to demonstrate its efficacy.

"Natural" or **alternative treatments** describe any treatment that has not been scientifically documented or identified as safe or effective for a certain medical condition. Examples of alternative treatments include acupuncture, yoga, herbal remedies, aromatherapy, biofeedback, and many others. In considering an alternative treatment, as with any scientifically documented treatment, one should consider the risks versus the benefits of such a treatment. If a particular procedure has no specific, direct risks associated with it, an important risk is potentially delayed treatment of the depression. For a mild depression, this risk may not be too great, but for a more severe depression with suicidal thoughts, it could be a fatal risk.

Other risks include loss of money on an ineffective treatment, the use of a treatment that is not standardized nor required to conform to specific regulations, and frustration when hopes of a unique treatment are not realized.

Herbal remedies are a popular natural choice for treatment of many conditions. A common assumption about these natural treatment choices is that they are safe because they are natural. Although herbs are found in nature, as with man-made chemicals, herbs have a specific chemical structure that also alters the body chemistry. As such, there can be significant side effects from such compounds as well. Some of these side effects can be life threatening. For example, there have been many cases of liver failure from use of kava supplements around the world. In many cases, the problem per se is not that there are side effects; it is that the herbal treatments are not regulated as to either their safety or efficacy. If a specific treatment is known to be effective, one may be willing to take certain risks for relief. Without known efficacy, however, it is not possible to make an informed decision about the risks from exposure. A lack of regulation also means that supplements available in the store are not rigorously tested for purity or quantity of the active compound in question. Individuals who sell these treatments may act as experts but have not necessarily obtained any specialized training or certification either. It is important to keep these issues in mind when undertaking an alternative treatment so that fully informed decisions about treatment can be made. If it is decided an alternative treatment should be tried, it is important to communicate this information with a doctor. Herbal treatments in particular may interact with other medications, making it especially important to do so.

50. Will diet or exercise help with my mood?

Anne's comment:

My husband has found a regular exercise regimen to be an important contribution to feeling well. It helps him to deal with stress and to maintain his weight, which might otherwise be adversely affected by his medication.

Depression is not caused by problems with diet, although some believe that a balanced diet would leave one less predisposed to difficulties handling stress and thus possibly any mood conditions that result from that stress. Problems with sleep as well are not considered causes of depression but can predispose someone to depressive symptoms when chronically under rested. Evidence exists for reduced concentration and irritability in persons with less then 6 hours of sleep per night. In individuals with manic depression, sleep hygiene is an important component of treatment, as reduced sleep can sometime trigger a manic episode in a susceptible individual.

Recent research has shown the effects of exercise on mood and anxiety. Although the medical benefits of exercise are well known, the psychological benefits are less understood. Adults who regularly exercise report lower rates of depression and anxiety than the general population. Studies of the effect of exercise on depression have demonstrated positive results. There are many theories as to how exercise improves mental health. Exercise causes changes in levels of serotonin, norepinephrine, and dopamine and causes the release of endorphins (which masks pain). It may reduce muscle tension, and adrenaline is released, counteracting the effects of stress. Psychologically too, exercise improves self-esteem, provides structure and routine, increases social contacts, and distracts from daily stress. Although the degree of impact that exercise has on depression needs more research, many good reasons exist for including regular exercise as part of a treatment plan for depression.

51. Why did my doctor recommend therapy if I am already taking medication?

Although therapy may be adequate alone for mild cases of depression, it is most optimal to be in therapy when taking medication. Studies have shown that therapy and medication together have the best efficacy. Although medication can treat your depression independently of therapy, it will not change environmental circumstances, will not change your coping skills, and will not change your personality or improve your self-esteem. Keeping in mind that depression is typically caused by a culmination of biological, psychological, and social factors, it makes good sense that addressing the psychological and social underpinnings of your depressive episode is warranted. Although you cannot change your "biology" or genes, you can use therapy to change other contributors to depression. Ideally, the risk then of future episodes can be reduced, as medication is generally not considered a life-long solution for managing depression, except in cases of more severe or chronic illness. Once in remission, an attempt to remove the medication is typically made. This is apt to be more successful when therapy has been or currently is in place.

52. My antidepressant is not helping. What happens next?

Anne's comment:

One of the most difficult aspects of treatment is the long period of trial and error to find the right types of medications and the right doses to treat my daughter's bipolar disorder effectively. It has taken almost 2 years to reach a point where she is relatively stable and not experiencing wild mood swings. Patience and perseverance have been part of the prescription, and the result is that she has been able to resume her life at college.

Anthony's comment:

You have to talk to your doctor. If feeling discouraged, consult with your doctor, as there are so many other choices to consider. My doctor changed my medication and said if it too doesn't work, we will try something else.

It can be disheartening when you do not feel better after a medication has been started. The pharmaceutical companies advertise their antidepressant medications in ways that suggest almost "miraculous" recovery. The reality is that the response rate to any given antidepressant tends to be approximately 60% to 70% in clinical trials. This means a good portion of individuals (more than 30%!) would not be expected to see improvement on the first medication tried. However, if a medication is not working, several factors first need to be considered: How long has the medicine been taken? Is the dose high enough? Is the medication being taken as prescribed?

It takes from 4 to 6 weeks (sometimes up to 8 weeks) for the full effect of an antidepressant to take place (after an adequate dose has been prescribed). Oftentimes, the dose of medication has not been optimized. As long as there are few or tolerable side effects, the dose can be pushed to the maximum recommended dosage (Appendix B). Your doctor may want to go past the typical maximum dose if you have no side effects and have partially responded to the treatment. However, in general, once the maximum dose has been prescribed for up to 6 weeks, and you have been taking it as prescribed, an adequate medication trial has occurred. If there is no improvement, a switch to another medication should be made. The change can even be within a class; for example, a lack of response to one SSRI does not mean the same will be true for another SSRI. If there is a partial response, your doctor may want to augment with another medication. Augmentation strategies generally involve using a medication with a different mechanism of action so that different neurotransmitter systems can come into play to help, similar to what cardiologists do when they prescribe antihypertensive medication to patients whose blood pressure remains elevated after an initial antihypertensive has been prescribed. Thus, if treatment with a given agent fails, management techniques include switches within a class, switches to another class, augmentation, the use of medications other than antidepressants, and ECT for more **refractory depression**.

Refractory depression

depressive illness that does not respond to multiple therapeutic interventions.

It is very important to be open with your doctor about your level of compliance with a given medication. It is not unusual for people to forget doses or skip doses for specific reasons. People often do not want to admit this to their doctor, as they think he or she will become upset with them. If you are having problems with taking your medication, it is extremely important for your doctor to know so that the two of you can discuss some of the barriers to taking it, such as side effects. A lack of efficacy is often due to regularly missed doses, and without this knowledge, other medications trials may be suggested unnecessarily.

53. Will the medication turn me into a zombie or make me look medicated?

Anne's comment:

Some of the medications that have been prescribed for my daughter have had a very sedating effect. When the effects of a particular medication are too disruptive, she has worked with her doctor to find more effective treatment. It is important for any patient to speak up and engage his or her doctor in a dialogue because the goal of treatment is to enable the patient to resume normal activities.

Looking "medicated" is often a reason that some people avoid treatment with antidepressants. Although some medications are used in psychiatric practice that can affect a person's state of alertness, perhaps making that person look robotic or overly sedated, antidepressants do not cause this. Sedation or sleepiness can sometimes occur as a side effect from some of the medications, but usually that can be avoided by changing the timing of the dose or switching to another medication. No one should be able to tell by your appearance that you are taking a medication for depression. In contrast, as depression can impair your concentration and cause decreased energy and fatigue, the use of antidepressant therapy is likely to make you more alert and less "robotic."

Some people worry that their personality will be changed by medication. Medication does not change a personality. Aside from the presence of side effects, you should experience no specific effects from an antidepressant. For some people, the lack of tranquilizing effects from an antidepressant sometimes leads to the conclusion that the medicine "is not doing anything." Antidepressants do not make you feel any differently or as if you have taken a medication. For someone who has been depressed for years (such as in dysthymic disorder), it may seem as if that is just a part of his or her personality so that once the depression is lifted one might wonder if his or her personality has changed. Similarly, some people believe that they will no longer experience sadness and thus not feel human. Sadness is in fact a normal emotion and is not supposed to be eliminated by antidepressant use. Some people do feel their emotions have dulled somewhat; if this occurs, it may simply mean a slightly lower dose of the medication is needed.

54. My medication is helping, but I have sexual side effects. What can I do?

Many antidepressants can have sexual side effects that range from decreased interest in sex to difficulty having an orgasm. Many individuals are too embarrassed to ask their doctor about these problems, but it is important to discuss such side effects and learn about your options. Depression itself can be a cause of reduced interest in sex, and thus, a determination first needs to be made as to whether the depression has remitted on the medication. If depressive symptoms are gone, then other considerations should also be made, such as what the baseline sexual functioning was before becoming depressed or before the treatment. As a group, SSRIs do have a very high incidence of sexual side effects associated with them. This can result in reduced compliance and thus reduced efficacy of the medication. Several options are available to address these effects. Sometimes, a "wait-and-see" approach is effective, as the negative effect may wane with time. Another option is to try another SSRI, which may not have the same effect for the individual, or to switch to a different class of antidepressant that does not typically cause sexual side effects. Antidepressants not typically associated with sexual side effects are as follows:

- Bupropion (Wellbutrin)
- Mirtazapine (Remeron)
- Nefazodone (Serzone)

As noted in Question 49, however, nefazodone has been implicated in some cases of liver failure and thus is not routinely prescribed anymore until other options have been exhausted. However, if the medication currently being taken is working, rather than take the risk of switching to another medication that may not be as effective, other types of medications can be prescribed in addition to the antidepressant that can counteract the effect that SSRIs have on sexual functioning. The different options should be discussed with your doctor, but current approaches include the use of sildenafil (Viagra), bupropion, and herbal remedies.

55. My doctor recommends medication for my depression. I am considering waiting to see whether my depression will go away without treatment.

Depression often occurs in cycles, and if an individual waits long enough, it may in fact remit without treatment. This may take months or longer, however. The risks of this approach are great: a loss of productivity in school/work, impaired relationships, family conflicts, financial problems, delays in development in children, and most significantly, suicide. Treatment of the depressive episode will greatly shorten its duration and enable you to participate in the community again sooner. In addition, research suggests that depression itself can have harmful effects on the brain. These effects may make you more susceptible to future depressive episodes, possibly more severe, in the future.

Untreated depression can have harmful effects on your physical health as well. Under stress, the body is less able to fight infection. Recovery from some physical illnesses may be adversely affected. Problems with sleep also impair the body's functioning, resulting in further loss of energy and difficulties in concentrating.

Depressed persons are at higher risk for drug and alcohol abuse, which can further worsen depressive symptoms and result in disability and problems with the law. Depressed persons are at risk of having problems in their relationships and getting a divorce. They may have difficulty developing strong **attachments** with their children.

Attachment

the psychological connection between a child and his or her caretaker.

Depressed children can have problems in their social and emotional development, making them at risk for further emotional problems in the future. Most significantly, untreated depression may increase the risk for suicide. Suicidal thoughts can gradually lead up to suicide attempts if the depression does not remit and feelings of hopelessness persist.

Treatment of depression is important for many reasons. A delay of its treatment may be as risky as delaying treatment for a multitude of medical conditions, such as heart problems, diabetes, high blood pressure, and cancer.

56. Can I take other medicines while I am on an antidepressant?

It is always important to inform any doctor you see of all medications that you are taking, including any herbal or over-the-counter supplements. Although many medications can be taken concurrently, the potential for reactions exists between many medications as well; thus, consideration must be given for this. Sometimes the potential reaction is minimal and may be due to additive side effects (e.g., sedating effects may combine). Other times, the presence of one medication can influence the elimination of the other medicine from the body, either allowing excessive accumulation or causing too rapid a depletion. Consequences can thus be toxicity or a lack of efficacy. The SSRIs have specific enzyme groups that **metabolize** the medication. Each SSRI has a different profile as to the enzymes involved in its own metabolism. MAOIs are generally contraindicated in combination with all other antidepressants because of the risk for **serotonin syndrome**, which can be fatal (although there are certain combinations that skilled clinicians can prescribe in a methodical way to minimize the risks). Serotonin syndrome occurs when an excess of serotonin exists in the central nervous system. Symptoms include tremor, confusion, incoordination, sweating, shivering, and agitation. Most SSRIs are contraindicated in combination with thioridazine (Mellaril) as well because of a risk of **cardiac toxicity**. SSRIs should be used cautiously in combination with sibutramine (Imitrex), commonly prescribed for migraine, because of a risk for serotonin syndrome. St. John's wort, an herbal preparation used for depression, should be avoided when on a prescribed antidepressant, also because of a potential risk for serotonin syndrome. Again, there are some circumstances when a psychiatrist will combine two SSRIs, for example, but this is typically done cautiously and under his or her guidance.

Metabolize
the process of breaking down a drug in the blood.

Serotonin syndrome
an extremely rare but life-threatening syndrome associated with the direct physiological effects of serotonin overload on the body.

Cardiac toxicity
damage that occurs to the heart or coronary arteries as a result of medication side effects.

As described in Question 42, MAOIs have very specific guidelines on foods to be avoided. Likewise, MAOIs can have significant interactions with other medications. As noted previously here, they are not to be combined with most other antidepressants. In fact, MAOIs have to be discontinued 2 weeks before a trial of another antidepressant, or the other antidepressant is to be discontinued for 2 weeks before initiating an MAOI. There are many over-the-counter medications to be avoided, such as pseudoephedrine and oxymetazoline; thus, it is important to check with your doctor and pharmacist before taking an over-the-counter medication while on an MAOI. This is sound policy with all medications, not just psychotropics.

57. My internist is prescribing an antidepressant. How do I know whether I should see a specialist? Should I see a psychopharmacologist?

A general practitioner of medicine can often adequately treat depression. There are situations, however, when a psychiatric consultation should be obtained. If there are co-morbid conditions such as anxiety or substance abuse, severe suicidal thinking, or complicated personality issues, a psychiatrist would be better equipped to manage the antidepressant treatment. In particular, the psychiatrist may be able to provide more frequent contacts and have longer sessions than the general practitioner typically has available. One problem that arises, however, when depression is treated by a general practitioner is that underdosing of medication is more common, as well as too short of a duration of treatment. Certainly if the depression is not responding to a prescribed treatment, consultation with a specialist is warranted as well.

Some individuals seek the services of a psychopharmacologist. The term can be somewhat misleading, as it implies a specialty in medication management of psychiatric conditions. In fact, all general psychiatrists are adequately trained in pharmacotherapy of mental disorders and need not be designated as psychopharmacologists. Some psychiatrists restrict their practice to medication management of mental disorders and thus are self-described as psychopharmacologists. Psychiatrists are available who develop more expertise in the management of certain conditions and use of some medications, by virtue of clinical experience and perhaps research in academic settings, and thus may take referrals from other psychiatrists (and mental health clinicians) for more refractory conditions. In general, however, seeking consultation from a general psychiatrist is usually appropriate for most emotional problems. Specialists may be sought within the field of psychiatry for treatment of children and adolescents (child and adolescent psychiatrist), older people (geriatric psychiatrist), people who are medically ill (consultation–liaison psychiatrist), and individuals with substance abuse (addiction psychiatrist).

58. Why do I need a mood stabilizer with my antidepressant if I am depressed but not manic?

"Mood stabilizer" has a variety of meanings attached to it. For the lay public, any medication that helps even one's moods, including the antidepressant medications, is a mood stabilizer. For most psychiatrists, mood stabilizer includes a class of medications that treat and prevent mania. These medications typically include anticonvulsant medications such as valproic acid and carbamazepine; atypical antipsychotic medications such as olanzapine, quetiapine, and risperidone; and lithium. However, the definition of a true mood stabilizer is a medication that treats and prevents both depression and mania. No true mood stabilizer by that definition exists. Perhaps lithium is the closest to meeting that definition, although it does not truly compare with antidepressants in effectively treating depression. Other antimanic medications that are never thought of as mood stabilizers include the antianxiety medications. At one time, alprazolam was used to treat certain forms of depression as well as anxiety and mania.

Thus, it is important to understand that when a psychiatrist adds a mood stabilizer to an antidepressant one needs to know exactly what class of agent is being prescribed and for what purpose. Many times patients may have associated symptoms with their depression (such as psychosis), and therefore, an atypical antipsychotic medication is an appropriate addition to the antidepressant. Still other patients may experience a great deal of anxiety and panic, in which case the addition of an antianxiety agent may be appropriate. Some patients may never have had a manic episode, but some of their symptoms and family history are strongly suggestive of an underlying bipolar disorder. Under these circumstances, the safest medication to prescribe may be a mood stabilizer alone, unless the depression is severe enough to warrant aggressive care, in which case the psychiatrist may prescribe an antidepressant with an anticonvulsant, lithium, or atypical antipsychotic as a preventative measure. Finally, some patients may achieve only a partial response to the antidepressant. When a partial response is achieved, the psychiatrist will typically add another medication to augment the primary medication's response rather than switch the medication altogether.

59. I have been prescribed an "off-label" medication. Does that mean that it is experimental?

"**Off label**" is used when a medication is used in a manner that is not Food and Drug Administration (FDA) approved. Does this mean the medication is experimental? No, absolutely not. This means simply that no studies have been submitted to the FDA for approval of the medication for that particular use. It does not mean that no studies have been done. Many studies may not have been submitted or may have been submitted and approved by European governments. It does not mean that the medication is not widely prescribed for a use other than what the FDA approved. It does not mean that doses under or over the recommended range approved by the FDA are neither effective nor safe. It does not mean that the medication is not safe in age groups younger or older than what the FDA approved. It merely means that when the company submitted the medication for approval to the FDA it submitted studies that specified a diagnosis, a dosage range, and an age group that their study subjects reflected.

Off-label
prescribing of a medication for indications other than those outlined by the Food and Drug Administration.

Drug research and development have a fascinating history. Psychiatric drugs are often discovered serendipitously. Most drugs have multiple effects on the body, and focusing on one particular action to the exclusion of another is often as much a matter of marketing as it is drug action. For example, the first antipsychotic medication was developed and tested by a trauma surgeon who was specifically interested in finding a medication that could prevent surgical shock, a condition with a high mortality rate at the time. It was only through clinical observation that it was discovered to have antipsychotic effects as well as a variety of other effects on the body. The company that originally introduced it to the United States did not believe that there would be a market for it as an antipsychotic and thus released it to the public as an antiemetic. Only through multiple physician-driven lectures were psychiatrists in the United States comfortable enough to try it on patients suffering from schizophrenia. Perhaps even odder is the fact that the first antidepressant effects were observed in medications developed to treat tuberculosis. Only later was it discovered that these medications inhibited, or blocked, monoamine oxidase, an enzyme that breaks down norepinephrine, serotonin, and dopamine at the synaptic cleft.

To call any particular medication an antihypertensive, an antipsychotic, an antidepressant, or an anticonvulsant is actually a misnomer and really reflects the target population that a particular medication is geared toward when released to the public, and not the broad range of effects of which the medication is capable. It also reflects the expense that the companies go through in order to obtain FDA approval. The FDA requires that each medication target a specific diagnosis in order to receive approval. This is a hugely expensive enterprise for one diagnosis, which is exponentially greater for multiple diagnoses. Therefore, it is unlikely drug companies will submit studies for approval for more than one or two diagnoses, unless they can see some return on investment. As a result, clinical practice is often very different from what the *Physicians' Desk Reference* (a standard reference of all FDA approved prescription medications) publishes. Clinical practice moves at a much faster pace than clinical trials and publications can keep up with. Although clinical trials are considered to be the definitive evidence of any particular medication's efficacy, astute clinical observations are what brought the biggest drug discoveries to the world and cannot be discounted simply because no study has yet to be published.

There are two broad reasons why off-label use makes sense in psychiatry. First, psychiatric diagnoses do not fit into the neat little categories that the DSM-IV-TR attempts to define. They generally have many overlapping symptoms. For example, anhedonia, or loss of interest, can be seen in a number of conditions that include depression, schizophrenia, and frontal lobe damage. Many psychiatrists believe that medications should be prescribed to target the particular neurochemicals underlying such specific symptoms regardless of the DSM diagnosis. Off-label use is practiced with a clear rationale for another reason as well. Human nature defies categories. Although there may be broad similarities between two individuals suffering from depression, it is doubtful that any one individual is suffering in exactly the same way as another from both a biochemical standpoint and a psychological standpoint. Thus, one may respond to one particular therapy or antidepressant and not another, and the reasons are due to the therapies' and antidepressants' biochemical differences, not their similarities. For these reasons, off-label use in psychiatry is more the rule than the exception. As an example of observation trumping scientific studies: a man sought out a cardiologist because he noticed getting palpitations from one particular brand of cola and not another. The cardiologist dismissed him outright. The man sought another cardiologist who agreed to perform a stress test after he ingested the different brands; sure enough, the man experienced premature ventricular beats with one particular brand of cola and not another. Never underestimate the power of one.

60. When is hospitalization necessary? What does it offer?

Hospitalization is the highest level of treatment. It is reserved for the most severe forms of depression (as well as other mental disorders). One criterion used for determining the necessity of hospitalization is the presence of suicidality. Having suicidal ideation does not automatically dictate a hospital stay but prompts an inquiry into the patient's level of risk to harm oneself (or others). Hospitalization may also be indicated if a person's functional impairment is so poor that he or she is unable to care adequately for himself or herself (e.g., unable to get out of bed and not eating). Most often, depressed individuals are willing to be hospitalized if recommended and thus do so voluntarily. Situations exist, however, when the physician believes hospitalization is necessary but the patient refuses. The physician then needs to decide whether the person should be admitted involuntarily. Criteria for involuntary admission varies from state to state, but it is generally not easy to admit someone against his or her will. Most states have mental hygiene laws in place to protect patient's rights. Typically, dangerousness to self or others is the criterion required to commit someone. Usually an appeal process is available to such a patient as well (see Question 89).

61. Can I drink wine with my antidepressant?

Generally speaking, because alcohol is a depressant, it is not advisable to drink alcohol of any kind when one is suffering from depression. With that being said, not everyone is on antidepressant medication for depression, and therefore, this advice may not pertain to you. However, many psychiatric illnesses have overlapping symptoms, particularly anxiety and depression. Just because your doctor may have prescribed the medication for anxiety rather than depression, the risk for depression is still higher than the general population, and thus, the need to abstain from alcohol remains good advice. Alcohol can also worsen anxiety and can lead to **dependence** in people suffering from anxiety because of its inherent antianxiety effects, causing some people to self-medicate with it.

Dependence
the body's reliance on a drug to function normally.

Is there any interaction between alcohol and antidepressants that could be dangerous if you still choose to drink alcohol? With some antidepressant medications such as MAOIs, the risk is serious, as the interaction with some forms of alcohol, particularly red wines, can lead to **malignant hypertension**, which is potentially life threatening. With TCAs, the risks are due to their sedative effects, which are additive to alcohol, and thus causing intoxication and its incumbent risks more readily. Finally, with the newer SSRIs, the additive effects are much less noticeable, as these medications are not found to be sedating or affecting cognition and

Malignant hypertension
elevated blood pressure that is acute and rapidly progressive with severe symptoms, including headache.

motor coordination adversely. It is best to be cautious if having wine or other alcohol in monitoring its effect on your mental status while on an antidepressant.

62. Are there long-term dangers to taking medication?

With the recent press regarding the alleged link between antidepressant medications and suicide (see Question 78), a fear has been that antidepressant medications are a form of mind control that can have permanent long-term effects on one's personality and one's mind. Such ideas are categorically false. The TCAs have been around for the longest period of time, approximately 50 years, and have never been associated with long-term dangers. The newer class of medications known as SSRIs has been around only since the introduction of Prozac in the late 1980s. Numerous studies have attempted to link them to long-term dangers such as cancer or other medical conditions aside from their psychologic effects. None of these studies has yet held up to any scrutiny. All of the studies linking SSRIs to suicidal behavior analyze data at the beginning of treatment and most likely represent an unidentified side effect that can be associated with suicidal behavior. Such side effects could be increasing anxiety and insomnia or an **extrapyramidal** side effect that cause patients to become uncomfortably restless (**akathisia**). Another factor that may be involved is the improvement in energy levels that often occurs before an improvement in mood, which may result in increased motivation and energy to act on suicidal desires. This is why close monitoring during the initial phase of treatment with these medications is imperative.

Extrapyramidal

the parts of the brain that are responsible for static motor control.

Akathisia

a subjective sense of inner restlessness resulting in the need to keep moving.

Although there are no documented long-term adverse effects from antidepressants, your doctor may want to monitor functioning of some organ systems with periodic blood work. The liver breaks down antidepressants, and thus, some people can rarely develop a mild impairment in liver functioning. In general, however, antidepressants as a group are not associated with long-term dangers.

Other medications may be used concurrently with antidepressants, such as anticonvulsants and antipsychotics that do have potential long-term effects on the liver or the kidney. In addition, antipsychotics have been associated with the development of a condition called **tardive dyskinesia**, which can be a permanent movement abnormality, usually of the mouth. This condition was much more common with older antipsychotic agents, but can rarely occur with the newer agents. Your doctor should monitor closely for such effects and should only continue the antipsychotic for the minimum duration that is necessary. For example, in psychotic depression, both an antidepressant and an antipsychotic are used in the treatment; however, the antipsychotic should be tapered and discontinued earlier than the antidepressant if possible.

Tardive dyskinesia
a late-onset involuntary movement disorder, often irreversible, typically of the mouth, tongue, or lips, a consequence of antipsychotic use, but less commonly observed with the newer atypical antipsychotics.

63. A lot of talk has happened in the press lately stating that antidepressants cause people to become suicidal or violent. What are the facts?

Violent acts directed toward oneself or others are very complex behaviors with multiple factors influencing them. Before discussing whether antidepressants cause people to become violent, it is important to understand what it means to state there is a causal link between these medications and violence. One normally thinks of cause in terms of simple physics such as a ball causing another ball to move when it strikes it. Obviously, this is not the same type of causal relationship that exists between antidepressants and violence. In the physical respect of causality, the only definitive thing that can be said of antidepressants is that they block a transporter pump, causing it to fail to reuptake a neurotransmitter at the synaptic cleft. How this causes an antidepressant effect after that is purely theoretical, although obviously based on sound scientific reasoning. If one reads the *Physicians' Desk Reference* regarding how antidepressants work, the text rightly states that it is unknown. Thus, even providing an explanation as to how antidepressants cause depression to lift is not definitively known.

Another type of causal relationship is the relationship that exists when thinking about what causes people to behave in certain ways. For example, hunger causes someone to eat or thirst causes someone to drink. These are apparently simple causal connections between feelings and acts. Other causal connections that are more complicated involve the issue of motives as in what is the motive behind someone committing a particular crime, such as revenge, jealousy, greed, etc. It is under these circumstances that people seek to understand the causal relationship between a violent act and the state of mind of the perpetrator just prior to committing the act. Typically, when one seemingly cannot find any rational motive behind a particular violent act, then the act is attributed to a mental illness. If someone is on drugs or alcohol or some other allegedly "mind-altering" medication, then those may be implicated as well. Although the mentally ill are far more likely to be victims of crimes rather than perpetrators of crimes, someone with mental illness tends to get more press when committing a crime. Most people with mental illnesses are on medication of some sort. Sorting out the causal link between a particular violent act and the underlying causes is similar to attempting to find the causal link between various genetic, physiological, and environmental factors that ultimately lead to disease but with the added complication of factoring in motive, intent, or one's state of mind. Therefore, all that can really be established are correlations. Currently, it appears that overall, since the introduction of SSRI antidepressants, rates of suicide have been decreasing. However, in many studies regarding particular SSRIs, it has been shown that an increased rate of suicide and suicide attempts occurs at the beginning of treatment. It is important to remember that these statistical analyses do not sort out the issues that are more pertinent to whether an SSRI will influence the odds that any one individual will attempt or succeed at suicide. For that, one must know the particular facts surrounding each particular attempt or completion.

Many possible reasons exist for there being increased violence during the initiation of antidepressant treatment. First, antidepressants have long been known to lead potentially to an increase in suicide during the initiation of treatment. This is attributed to the fact that there is generally an improvement in energy before there is an improvement in mood so that a depressed patient now has the drive to act on his or her suicidal thoughts. Second, it appears that SSRIs with shorter half-lives (i.e., SSRIs that are metabolized and eliminated by the body more rapidly) appear to have a stronger correlation than SSRIs with longer half-lives. This may be due to the fact that there is an association between half-life and the discontinuation syndrome one experiences when stopping these medications abruptly. The discontinuation syndrome can be extremely uncomfortable and anxiety provoking, prompting individuals to misinterpret their symptoms as a worsening of their depression. At this point, this relationship is purely speculative. Third, the antidepressants themselves have side effects associated with them, including agitation, restlessness, anxiety, insomnia, headaches, and indigestion. These side effects can be misinterpreted as a worsening of depression, even though they are not. Finally, in some rare patients, antidepressants may cause a switch into a manic state, during which there can be irritability and poor impulse control in the presence of suicidal or homicidal ideation.

Statistically speaking, the increased use of antidepressants in the population leads to an increased probability that people exposed to antidepressants will attempt or complete suicide merely by the fact that they would have acted on these thoughts whether they were on the antidepressants or not. If the entire population of the United States were given antidepressant medications and the rates of violent acts increased slightly during the year that they received them (violent acts have an annual statistical variability), the correlation between the medication and the acts would be 100%. This would have absolutely no meaning in terms of figuring out a causal link. Thus, at present, no clear causal links are established between antidepressant use and violence.

64. Why did my doctor prescribe an antipsychotic for me when I am just depressed?

Antipsychotic medications are often prescribed for patients suffering from psychotic symptoms resulting from their depression. Such symptoms often revolve around false beliefs that the patient deserves some horrible punishment for a minor transgression that the patient believes to be a major sin or crime. Antipsychotics specifically target those symptoms, thus relieving patients of those painful thoughts and feelings. With the introduction of newer antipsychotic medications, however, their use as augmenting agents to antidepressants even in the absence of psychosis has become a new option for psychiatrists.

The newer antipsychotic medications, often called atypical antipsychotics or **second-generation antipsychotics** (SGAs), were developed because of increasing concern regarding the risk of developing a severe, potentially irreversible movement disorder known as tardive dyskinesia. Patients suffering from mood disorders are at greater risk for developing this movement disorder than patients who suffer primarily from psychotic disorders. SGAs have reduced this risk dramatically. They are, as a result, generally safer to use than their predecessors, although recently, there have been growing concerns about their metabolic effects on the body, including the potential for weight gain, increased blood sugar, and increased cholesterol and lipids. Despite these concerns, they remain an effective strategy when patients are showing only a partial response to their antidepressant medication or have a history of

Second-generation antipsychotic

an antipsychotic with a profile of targeted brain receptors that differs from older antipsychotics.

bipolar disorder and need medication to prevent the possibility of mania while undergoing treatment with an antidepressant medication.

SGAs include clozapine (Clozaril), quetiapine (Seroquel), olanzapine (Zyprexa), risperidone (Risperdal), ziprasidone (Geodon), and aripiprazole (Abilify). The reason that SGAs appear to have a broader spectrum of effectiveness than their predecessors has to do with the multiple neurotransmitter effects that these medications have, particularly on the neurotransmitter serotonin. As a result, these medications appear to improve anxiety and insomnia, enhance attention and concentration, and provide some antidepressant as well as clear antimanic treatment and prevention. Psychiatrists use them for all of these reasons, usually at doses lower than needed for psychotic symptoms. Most of these uses are off label, but again, that does not mean that they are experimental. Many studies support their use in this manner. Again, it is important to remember that because a physician is prescribing an antipsychotic (or an antidepressant or anticonvulsant, etc.), he or she does not necessarily believe that you are psychotic (or depressed or suffering from epilepsy, etc.). It is always important to ask the physician about the rationale behind prescribing any medication.

65. How does generic medication differ from trade names?

The generic name of a medication is the international scientific name for the molecule that constitutes the active form of the medication. The company that develops the medication then applies for a patent and obtains exclusive rights to sell the medication. It then gives the medication a trade name, which can change from country to country and from its intended use. For example, the medication with the generic name paroxetine is marketed under the trade name Paxil in the United States and Seroxat in the United Kingdom. The medication with the generic name bupropion is used as an antidepressant under the trade name Wellbutrin and as a smoking cessation medication under the name Zyban. The medication with the generic name fluoxetine is used under the trade name Prozac as an antidepressant and as Sarafem, a medication prescribed by obstetricians for women suffering from premenstrual symptoms. Once a medication goes off patent, other companies obtain the right to make and sell it. At this point, generic forms of the medication that may be less expensive become available. These medications are sold under their generic names. As physicians first know the original form of the medication by its trade name, the physicians often continue to write prescriptions under that name. By law, pharmacies must fill the prescription with the less expensive form of the medication unless the physician specifically indicates to the pharmacy not to substitute. As a result, the filled prescription will come back to the patient under the generic name rather than the trade name.

Are there differences between generic medications and medications under the trade name? The active ingredients of the medication are identical. The "fillers" or inactive ingredients making up the rest of the medication may differ. There may also be more percentage variations between the amounts of active ingredients from pill to pill in generic medications than in trade medications, as the requirements for quantity control are more stringent with trade medications than with generic medications. These differences are so minute as to be negligible, and with repeated dosing, the differences cancel each other. Patients have noticed differences initially in the way they feel when they switch from a trade to a generic medication, but this feeling is lost over time as the medication levels achieve a steady state in the person.

66. *Are antidepressants prescribed for reasons other than depression?*

The term antidepressant is actually a misnomer (see Question 59). Most psychoactive medications have multiple effects, and the decision to label a particular medication an antidepressant, an anticonvulsant, an antipsychotic, or an anxiolytic is often as much a matter of marketing as it is because of the drug's clinical effects. The newer class of antidepressants called SSRIs, for example, were originally developed and designed in the 1960s as potential antihypertensive medications. TCAs may have been marketed as antacids if not for the discovery of cimetidine (Tagamet), the first antihistamine antacid discovered.

Neuropathic pain

pain secondary to an abnormal state, such as degeneration, of nerves.

Antidepressant medications have multiple properties that are used by different physicians to target specific symptoms with which their patient's present. For example, neurologists have long been using TCAs to prevent migraine headaches, and endocrinologists have been using them to manage **neuropathic pain** associated with diabetes. Recently, rheumatologists have found success with SSRIs to target the symptoms associated with fibromyalgia. One of the most effective medications to manage irritable bowel syndrome has been paroxetine. Aside from depression, the list of conditions that respond to antidepressant medications is fairly long. It includes most anxiety disorders, but especially, generalized anxiety disorder, panic disorder, obsessive–compulsive disorder, and posttraumatic stress disorder. However, they are also indicated in eating disorders as well as **somatoform** disorders. Internists use them extensively to treat insomnia, chronic pain disorders, and chronic fatigue syndrome. Obstetricians use them to manage dysmenorrhea and perimenopausal symptoms (see Tables 10 and 11 for conditions that antidepressants can treat).

Somatoform
pertaining to conditions with physical symptoms thought due to psychological factors.

Table 10 Indications for the use of Antidepressants

Mood disorders
Anxiety disorders
Sleep disorders
Chronic pain disorders
Chronic fatigue disorder
Adjunctive therapy for other functional somatic syndromes

Table 11 Functional Somatic Syndromes

Fibromyalgia
Chronic back pain
Irritable bowel syndrome
Primary dysmenorrhea
Myofascial pain
Chronic tension headache
Temporomandibular joint disease (TMJ)
Non-cardiac chest pain
Multiple chemical sensitivity

Functional
generally referring to a symptom or condition that has no clearly defined physiological or anatomical cause.

PART FIVE

Associated Conditions

I have been diagnosed with depression and anxiety. How is the combination of conditions treated?

My spouse is drinking a lot of alcohol lately. My friend thinks he might be self-medicating. What does that mean?

Why is my doctor telling me that I need treatment for my addiction when I thought treating the depression would solve my problem?

More . . .

67. I have been diagnosed with depression and anxiety. How is the combination of conditions treated?

Anne's comment:

One of my children was treated with antidepressants for 9 months before revealing that he had been experiencing anxiety for a long time and had hoped that the antidepressant medication, which improved his depression, would also assuage his anxiety. In fact, his anxiety had become acute, and he experienced tremendous relief with the addition of antianxiety medication to his medication regimen.

Anxiety is a condition that commonly occurs with depression. Some anxiety conditions, such as social phobia, panic disorder, and generalized anxiety disorder, may predispose someone for the development of a depressive disorder because of the significant impact that severe anxiety can have on a person's functioning. Likewise, depression can also trigger the onset of an anxiety disorder. The treatment for both conditions is often very similar, and both conditions can often be addressed with the same medication or type of therapy. The SSRIs are a very useful treatment for many anxiety disorders and thus are ideal in persons who suffer from both anxiety and depression. As in the treatment of depression, the SSRIs can take a few weeks to have their full benefit for anxiety. Also, higher dosing of SSRIs is often needed to address anxiety, even after depressive symptoms have remitted on a given dosage. Because of the delayed onset of relief, short-term treatment of anxiety is sometimes necessary, particularly in cases of severe anxiety that results in significant impairment. In the short-term, anxiety is better treated with benzodiazepines, which typically provide rapid relief of anxious symptoms but are controlled substances that can be habit forming and thus are not generally recommended for long-term use. Buspirone is a nonaddictive antianxiety medication that is used for generalized anxiety. It may be a better choice in persons with substance abuse histories or active substance abuse. Buspirone does not offer immediate relief of anxiety. It also requires 4 to 6 weeks before a full effect is seen. Concurrent anxiety can result in refractory depression, and thus, it is important that untreated anxious symptoms are addressed if there seems to be little response to an antidepressant.

Psychotherapy is a very important treatment for anxiety. Cognitive–behavioral therapy in particular has been demonstrated in studies to have beneficial results for a variety of anxiety conditions. Although medications are very effective in reducing severe anxiety, significant residual symptoms are often left, and therapy helps to reduce these further. A combination of therapy and medication is typically the best treatment approach for a variety of anxiety disorders, such as generalized anxiety disorder, panic disorder, social anxiety disorder, and obsessive–compulsive disorder.

68. My spouse is drinking a lot of alcohol lately. My friend thinks he might be self-medicating. What does that mean?

Individuals with depression may abuse alcohol or drugs in a misguided effort to feel better. Alcohol can initially give the impression of improving one's mood, but in actuality, alcohol is a depressant. Likewise, the use of drugs to get "high" is usually followed by a "crash," during which the mood becomes sad or despondent. Sometimes depression is caused by the alcohol or drug abuse itself and will remit when abstinence is achieved. Oftentimes, depression precedes the alcohol or drug use, and people turn to these substances in an effort to feel better. Typically, however, feeling better really just means being "numb" or deadened to the depressed feelings. Treatment of the depression rarely may result in achievement of abstinence, which will depend on the stage of substance abuse. If the individual has become dependent (addicted) to the alcohol or drugs, then concordant substance abuse treatment will likely be necessary as well. As long as the person is addicted to alcohol or drugs, recovery from depression will be limited. In fact, substance abuse is a problem that needs to be considered if someone is refractory to treatments for depression. Seeing a person who specializes in treatment of addictions would also be helpful, as there are different forms of therapeutic interventions often needed in persons who have addiction. In addition, there are specialized treatment programs for persons with both depression and substance abuse.

69. Why is my doctor telling me that I need treatment for my addiction when I thought treating the depression would solve my problem?

Anne's comment:

A large percentage of bipolar patients are dual diagnosis, meaning that they have addiction issues in addition to their bipolar disorder. It is extremely important for dual-

diagnosis patients to receive ongoing treatment for both aspects of their illness. Relapsing into alcohol or drugs will cause the bipolar patient to destabilize, and an entire cycle of healing will have been negated.

Patients with a combination of addiction and depression are at higher risk for suicide, homicide, poor compliance, relapse, and greater hospitalization rates. Although some evidence exists to support the concept that many patients use substances to "self-medicate" an underlying depression, no evidence exists showing that antidepressant medication leads to abstinence. Although the "self-medication hypothesis" may seem right for some individuals, once an addiction develops, it takes on a life of its own. It is unlikely that medicating it away can conquer addiction. Also, if you continue to use drugs or alcohol while receiving antidepressant medication, the medication is rendered essentially ineffective. Thus, depression cannot be effectively treated without also treating the addiction.

70. How are alcoholism and depression connected?

A clear link exists between addiction and depression. The rates of depression are three times higher in male addicts and four times higher in female addicts than in the general population, and a third of all depressed patients suffer from an addiction. Men typically develop a substance abuse disorder first, whereas women typically develop a mood disorder first. The link between these conditions has biological, psychological, and social roots. Biologically, many addictive substances are depressants, whereas many other addictive substances when withdrawn cause depression. Additionally, both addiction and depression run together in families, placing individuals at risk genetically. Psychologically, certain personalities are prone to addiction and depression. People who have difficulty with impulse control, who are quick to anger, and who are abrupt seem to be more prone to addiction, perhaps as an attempt to help modulate their feelings. Unfortunately, these addictions are only transiently beneficial and generally backfire. Alternatively, people who are shy or reserved and who become very anxious in social settings are more prone to depression and addiction as well, again because they often use substances as a way of trying to feel more comfortable "in their own skin" as well as around others. Socially, people who struggle with depression and addiction find themselves socially isolated and unable to keep a job. Social isolation, job loss, and loss of access to healthcare and housing can lead people to further worsening of symptoms of depression and addiction.

71. I have not been able to sleep well or concentrate at work since being mugged 3 months ago. Could I be depressed?

Psychological trauma, which occurs in response to a physical threat to life or bodily integrity, is one of many risk factors for depression. It can be exposure to military combat, violent assault, child abuse, domestic violence, accidents, or natural disasters. Witnessing a traumatic event or hearing about a trauma from a loved one can also cause trauma. Nearly everyone who experiences a traumatic incident will suffer from some of the symptoms of traumatic stress. However, only between 7% and 25% will suffer enough symptoms to meet the criteria for acute traumatic stress disorder. The range depends on the type of trauma experienced. Of those who develop acute traumatic stress disorder, 80% will go on to develop posttraumatic stress disorder. Not everyone exposed to severe trauma will develop posttraumatic stress disorder. Risk factors that confer a vulnerability to posttraumatic stress disorder include the following:

- A psychiatric history
- A history of previous trauma
- Low intelligence
- Limited social supports
- Separation from parents in childhood, or early parental divorce
- A family history of depression or anxiety

As a general rule, all psychiatric disorders, particularly posttraumatic stress disorder, are more apt to become chronic the longer symptoms persist and may take longer to abate with treatment. The rates of depression and alcoholism are extremely high among those suffering from posttraumatic stress disorder, and left untreated, they essentially "fuel the posttraumatic stress disorder fire" through continued depression and substance abuse. Posttraumatic stress disorder and major depression have a number of symptoms in common, and major depression frequently develops secondary to posttraumatic stress disorder. It is important to be evaluated as soon as possible. Psychotherapy is an essential part of the treatment, and medication may be necessary, particularly if there are co-morbid conditions.

72. Since returning from active duty overseas, my husband is having nightmares, is afraid to go out, and is quieter than his usual self. Is this posttraumatic stress? Will it go away?

Re-experiencing
the phenomenon of having a previous lived experience vividly recalled and accompanied by the same strong emotions one originally experienced.

Numbing
the psychologic process of becoming resistant to external stimuli so that previously pleasurable activities become less desirable.

Posttraumatic stress disorder is a common combat casualty for many soldiers returning from war. It is associated with three primary symptoms that persist for longer than a month after a traumatic event: (1) **re-experiencing**, such as flashbacks or nightmares or intense memories; (2) hyperarousal, such as jumping at noises one used to ignore; and (3) **numbing**, such as an inability to feel pleasure and a tendency to isolate.

After the intensity of combat where life is "black and white," civilian life appears drab and overly complicated, further adding to the distress and isolation. There is a strong possibility that posttraumatic stress disorder will lead to substance abuse and depression if left untreated. In some studies, as many as 52% develop alcohol abuse or dependence, and 47% develop depression. In a recent study of U.S. soldiers returning from Iraq, approximately 16% said that they were experiencing symptoms of depression and anxiety associated with posttraumatic stress disorder. The highest rates of symptoms result from being shot at, being ambushed, receiving artillery, shooting or directing fire at the enemy, or seeing human remains. Natural disasters are less prone to result in posttraumatic stress disorder than man-made disasters.

There is no absolutely clear understanding of why some soldiers are at greater risk for developing posttraumatic stress disorder than others. Aside from the type of exposure as mentioned previously, it appears that reservists are more prone than careerists. Additionally, premorbid personality and mental health factors may play a role, as well as prior exposure to traumatic incidents. Finally, cultural and political factors as well as social supports have impact on the soldiers. The lack of clear identification of friend from foe during their tour of duty, their sense of society's attitude toward them and the war after returning from their tour, and the support system available to them after return have significant influence on soldiers' vulnerability to mental illness. Unfortunately, many, if not most, soldiers will not admit to having a problem or seek help. They have been trained to "suck it up," and any admission of emotional problems related to their duty is an admission of weakness in the face of their responsibility. Those who usually do admit to the problems are ostracized and accused of weakness. Question 71 noted that the earlier your spouse gets into treatment, the better the chance for a positive outcome.

73. I am not getting any better despite numerous medication trials. My doctor says I have a personality disorder that medication will not treat and recommends more intensive therapy. What does he mean by that?

As mentioned in previous questions concerning the DSM-IV-TR, the diagnosis of a personality disorder is a complicated and controversial issue. As noted in Question 4, the DSM-IV-TR divides different diagnoses into Axis I, or major mental illnesses, and Axis

II, or personality disorders. Axis III is for coding of medical conditions. The notion that personality disorders are separate from major mental illnesses stems, in part, from an understanding that there is a difference between the changing states of mood and thinking over time, and those personality traits that seem a part of what makes a person who he or she is. For example, there are people who are naturally outgoing, gregarious, and quick to try new things. Quite the opposite, there are those who are shy, reserved, and uncomfortable in new and unfamiliar situations and environments. Most people have some elements of both traits that vary with particular situations but the traits are generally of an enduring quality. But whether or not one is shy or outgoing by nature, depression can plague both types. Consider some well-known celebrities who have recently spoken in public of their struggles with depression. These celebrities are generally gregarious people who seem to have everything going for them so it comes as a surprise when they speak of their depression and its treatment. One naturally thinks of a depressive personality when one thinks of someone struggling with depression. But depression can affect anyone. The treatment fortunately restores one back to his or her "old self," that can include all the idiosyncratic behaviors or "quirks" of personality that define who one is as a person.

When people gossip about one another, sharing particular stories about their friends, bosses, or colleagues and how they are as people, the general themes outlined from those stories characterize the personality profiles of the people and how best to act around them based on those profiles. The attempt to classify personality has a rich and complicated history that remains unfinished, including psychoanalysis, with its narrative approach, as well as psychometrics with various paper and pencil tests. But personality has been difficult to classify as most people have personalities that do vary somewhat with their circumstances and the people around them. Still, personality as a concept has enormous utility, as gossip continues to allow people to negotiate the complicated interpersonal terrain of their lives. The definition of personality can be likened to the definition of pornography, where defining it may be difficult, but one knows it when they see it. The DSM-III and its various editions since, as a manual of psychopathology, has attempted to classify personality when it goes wrong, or when it leads to distress or disability. The DSM-IV-TR defines a personality disorder as, "an enduring pattern of inner experience and behavior that deviates markedly from the expectations of the individual's culture, is pervasive and inflexible, has an onset in adolescence or early adulthood, is stable over time, and leads to distress or impairment" (pg. 685).

The various personality disorders are broken down into three broad categories, known among clinicians as clusters A, B, and C. These can best be described as "odd" for cluster A, "dramatic" for cluster B, and "anxious" for cluster C. Each adjective gives a general "flavor" for the various personality disorders subsumed by the cluster. Each cluster has three to four specific personality disorders associated with the cluster. Most of us have traits that we can easily identify in ourselves associated with each cluster. That is because the three clusters pretty much capture all personality types that exist in the world in broad-brush strokes. But it is only when the traits become so fixed that they lead to dangerous or self-defeating behavior that they are labeled disordered.

Medication has traditionally not been an effective treatment for personality disorders. Instead, intensive psychotherapy has been the recommended intervention. While this rule generally remains in effect, recently, particularly with the introduction of SSRIs, some personality traits have appeared to respond to medication. This has been particularly true for traits that involve extremely shy, reserved individuals traditionally known as having avoidant personality disorders but are now often diagnosed under Axis I with social phobia. As a result, the boundary between Axis I and Axis II has become blurred, offering new hope for individuals previously thought to benefit only from intensive outpatient therapy. There are now, however, challenging ethical questions regarding the use of medications to alter personality "cosmetically" along the same lines that plastic surgery cosmetically alters physical appearance.

While this example illustrates the advancement psychopharmacology has made in the past decade, unfortunately most personality disorders are not as responsive to medication interventions as therapy. In particular, for the cluster B disorder, borderline personality disorder, dialectical behavior therapy in addition to medication remains the standard of care. Borderline personality disorder remains one of the most difficult and devastating personality disorders to diagnose and treat. It is accompanied by inner feelings of rejection sensitivity, rapidly shifting moods, which are extreme and directly related to good or bad news received, and severe self-injurious behavior with frequent impulsive suicide attempts. Even with mood stabilizing and antidepressant medication, the behaviors can continue to plague individuals and their families with frequent hospitalizations and an increased frustration for everyone involved. Many times these individuals have multiple psychiatric diagnoses that can be as much an attempt to stabilize them with medication as a sense of frustration regarding lack of response to multiple treatment interventions. While such a patient may view recommendations for intensive therapy as another example of abandonment, it is exactly what is required to have a chance at getting better. Oftentimes more than one care provider working in a team that will provide both medication and therapy is a useful treatment approach, and any recommendation short of including intensive therapy would not be in the patient's best interest.

PART SIX

Special Populations

Do children get depressed?

The guidance counselor at school thinks that our teenage daughter is depressed. She spends a lot of time in her room. Is this normal teen behavior?

More . . .

74. Do children get depressed?

Anne's comment:

One of the first clues to our child's depression was profoundly irritable and unreasonable behavior. Despite therapy, the depression worsened, and academic problems and the inability to concentrate became pronounced. With aggressive treatment with a course of antidepressants and continued therapy, our child's mood stabilized, and academic performance returned to normal. The intervening months of waiting for the medication to take effect were the most challenging. We were very careful to remain positive and encouraging during the months that academic grades tumbled.

Children and adolescents can suffer from depression, as well as many other mental conditions once believed to afflict only adults. The risk of untreated depression in children and adolescents is the same as for those in adults, but social–emotional development, as well as academic progress, may fall behind because of the impairment in functioning. Some differences in criteria are used to diagnose depression in children, but essentially, the presenting symptoms are the same as in adults. Children do not always exhibit depressed mood but may be irritable instead. Depression often manifests with behavioral problems rather than a withdrawal from others. Behavioral problems in children that may be associated with depression include fighting with peers, increased defiance toward adults, a decline in grades, disruptive behavior in school, or school avoidance.

It was once believed that children and adolescents rarely suffered from significant depression. Teenage years are often believed to be tumultuous by nature and a sufficient explanation for problems of moodiness, oppositional behavior, school troubles, etc. Studies that have looked into the past of depressed adults have found that many adults first suffered from depression as adolescents. At any time, 10% to 15% of children and adolescents suffer from some symptoms of depression. Because of the adverse effect on social and emotional development, it is very important to treat depression in these age groups. Depressed adolescents are at a higher risk for substance abuse and early sexual experimentation, school failure, running away, and legal problems. Suicide is the third leading cause of death in adolescents. The family is often in crisis when a child suffers from an emotional disorder, putting a strain on siblings and parents. Parents may have to take extra time off from work to address school problems and to tend to the emotional and behavioral issues. They may not be as available for siblings who might feel neglected. Failure to recognize depression in children and adolescents is fraught with significant risks for everyone in the family. Depression is a treatable illness in children and adolescents and should be taken very seriously.

75. The guidance counselor at school thinks that our teenage daughter is depressed. She spends a lot of time in her room. Is this normal teen behavior?

It is often believed that adolescence is characterized by turmoil and significant distress. In fact, most teenagers do not experience high levels of turmoil and undergo transitions into adulthood relatively smoothly. As adolescents begin to establish their own identities, they begin to pull back emotionally from their parents. They may isolate in their room more frequently and may refuse to spend time with their parents. As a result, many parents do not know how their teenager is coping with and processing events around them. When locked in their room, teenagers may appear to be acting as any normal teen would. Although many depressed adolescents present with behavioral difficulties that are obvious to their guardians, many teens suffer silently, without showing their feelings. Parents may not be aware that a problem exists. At school, an adolescent may talk openly with the guidance counselor or teacher, perhaps as a way of getting help without admitting to the parents that there is a problem. Whenever there is a change in behavior, there should be consideration of emotional problems as a cause, rather than strictly assuming that it is "hormonal" or typical for teenagers.

76. What are the risks for suicide in children and adolescents?

Suicide is a very real risk for depressed youth. Suicide is the third leading cause of death in teenagers. A study by the Centers for Disease Control and Prevention of high school students yielded information that nearly 20% of teens had seriously considered suicide and that more than 1 in 12 had made a suicide attempt in the previous year. Male teens are more likely to kill themselves, whereas more females attempt suicide. The majority of teen suicides are with guns. Children also can have suicidal ideation but are less apt to make attempts the younger they are.

Risk factors for suicide include the following:

- Previous suicide attempts
- Depression
- Alcohol or substance abuse
- A family history of psychiatric illness
- Stressful circumstances
- Access to guns
- An exposure to other teens who have committed suicide

Stressful life events tend to be higher in children and adolescents who attempt suicide and may include loss of family members because of death or separation, physical or sexual abuse, frequent arguing in the home, or witnessing violence. Youth who are grappling with their sexual identity are at particularly high risk for suicide. Suicidal youth tend to have poor social adjustment and are lacking adequate social supports.

Some depressed adolescents engage in the self-injurious behavior of cutting themselves without the specific intention of killing themselves. This is more typical in persons who experience a chronic emptiness and "emotional numbness." The pain from cutting is described as a relief because the physical pain detracts from the emotional pain. Such behaviors are a sign that help is needed and are typically seen in depression when occurring in adolescence, but they are also a feature in some personality disorders in adults. Although those who engage in self-injurious behaviors do not necessarily intend to kill themselves, accidental death is a risk as well as the development of permanent scarring. Oftentimes, the cutting behavior is transient, occurring during particularly stressful periods (e.g., loss of relationship), and dissipates with the development of better coping skills and improved impulse control.

77. *What is the treatment approach for children and adolescents?*

Anne's comment:

One of the most important aspects in treating our child's depression was participating in weekly therapy with him until his condition became more stable. This facilitated the therapist in assessing our son's progress and helped us to communicate better and be more supportive as he struggled through the worst stages of the illness. It was an invaluable tool for all of us during a time of crisis.

The treatment of children and adolescents must first begin with a comprehensive evaluation by a qualified practitioner. It is important that the treatment provider has experience with this population or better yet has specialty training with this population. The evaluation tends to encompass more areas of query than do adult evaluations, with full developmental history and family history obtained, and school functioning assessed and contrasted with home functioning. As in adults, other conditions must be considered and excluded before diagnosing depression. Once diagnosed with depression, a treatment plan might address the following areas:

- Individual
- Medical
- Family
- School
- Legal

Individual needs can be addressed with psychotherapy. Cognitive–behavioral therapy and interpersonal therapy approaches have been studied and found to be effective in adolescent depression. Children and adolescents can benefit from other psychotherapeutic approaches as well. Group therapy should be considered if concerns exist about social development. In addition to individual psychotherapy, work with children and adolescents often needs some level of family work, either with the parents or with siblings. As members of a family system, dynamics between the child and others cannot always be effectively addressed in individual work alone. Problems with behavior may require enhancement of parenting skills. Psychoeducation of family members too may be needed to help them understand the patient's illness.

Medically, the use of somatic treatments, such as an antidepressant medication, may be recommended for depression in a child or adolescent. All children and adolescents should have medical clearance through their pediatrician to exclude any underlying medical conditions. Depending on the severity of the depression, an antidepressant may or may not be recommended. It is more commonplace to attempt a trial at therapy alone in children and adolescents first in contrast to adults. However, if progress is slow or if symptoms worsen, a consultation for medication can then be sought.

Educational needs are also assessed in children and adolescents. Depression can cause academic delays and may be associated with co-morbid learning disabilities. If significant academic problems exist, a board of education assessment may be needed to determine the most appropriate educational setting. Most states mandate that appropriate educational services be made available to minors with emotional and/or behavioral problems, which may consist of smaller classroom settings, nonpublic school placement, day treatment programs, or even residential treatment settings.

The legal needs of a child also have to be considered in the evaluation process. As a minor, the parent or guardian will make the final decision regarding the treatment intervention. Older adolescents, however, do have some say regarding their treatment. It is best if they are in agreement to a medication because they cannot be forced to take a medication against their will. Other legal issues to consider are custody issues and the need for family court involvement or state involvement.

78. What are the risks of treating my teenager with an antidepressant?

Although various antidepressant medications are effective in treating adults with depression, these medications may not be as effective in treating children and adolescents. Monitoring of medication therapy must be done very closely.

A general paucity of scientific data is available regarding medication use in children and adolescents. In years past, it was often presumed that medications worked in young people the same as in adults. Clinical trials rarely included persons under the age of 18 years. FDA approval for most psychotropic medications is strictly applicable to adult populations. The use of many antidepressants in children and adolescents is therefore considered "off label." Before the development of SSRIs, children and adolescents were rarely treated with antidepressants. The tricyclics and MAOIs that were available had potentially harmful side effect profiles that outweighed the benefit of the treatment. This was in part due to the fact that clinical studies in persons under 18 did not demonstrate antidepressants to be more effective than placebo. When SSRIs entered the market, however, because of their better safety profile, prescriptions for antidepressants in children and adolescents increased dramatically. There was clearly a need for safe, effective treatments, as in adults, untreated depression has serious adverse outcomes. In recent years, studies of SSRIs have been conducted in children and adolescent populations, with efficacy demonstrated in some. One observation from SSRI studies (that was also noted in the early studies using tricyclics) was the presence of a relatively high placebo response rate. Adolescents may benefit from the supportive contact with the treatment provider and thus "respond" to the placebo. Talk therapy is clearly a necessary part of treating depression in children and adolescents, even if on medication. Currently, the only SSRI with FDA approval for treatment of depression in pediatric populations is fluoxetine. Sertraline and fluvoxamine have FDA approval for treatment of pediatric obsessive–compulsive disorder.

Antidepressant therapy for children and adolescents can be a difficult decision for many parents who are wary of starting a medication for emotional or behavioral problems. Many teens too are wary of taking medication for fear of being recognized as "crazy." As with adults, the risk of taking medication must be balanced against the risk of forgoing medication treatment. When it comes to children and adolescents, understanding the risks of medication can be more difficult, however, because of the scarcity of scientific studies, as well as the evidence for higher placebo responses than in adults. Certainly, the severity of the depression must be taken into account when weighing the risks. The more severe the depression is the slower the response might be to a talk therapy intervention alone. In addition, there have been recent concerns about the possibility of increased suicidal thinking in children and adolescents who are prescribed SSRIs. A recent analysis by the FDA of all the studies of newer antidepressants showed a rate of suicidal behaviors in 3% to 4% of children and adolescents with depression who took an antidepressant and a rate of 1% to 2% of those taking a placebo (inactive pill). Of note, there were no deaths by suicide in any of the studies. Also, there was no difference in the rate of suicidal behavior for those being treated with an antidepressant for an anxiety disorder. The results of the analysis have prompted the FDA to require a warning on all antidepressants regarding the risk of increased suicidal behavior (thoughts or actions) when used in children and adolescents. While this can be disconcerting for any parent, it is important to keep in mind that the risk for suicide in untreated depression is approximately 15%. Reasons for the increased rate while on medication may be due to some of the factors described in Question 63, but it is not understood at this time. What is important to keep in mind is the necessity for close monitoring. As in adults, depression is a condition that is associated with suicidality. Whether on an antidepressant or not, patients need to be closely monitored for the onset of such symptoms or worsening of existing symptoms. Keeping the data in mind, in contrast to fears of increased suicidal tendencies, data from around the world actually document that the suicide rate among teenagers has dropped concordant with increased prescribing of SSRIs for depression.

79. Our child has been diagnosed with diabetes. She is having behavioral problems at school and home and is angry all of the time. What can we do?

Children and adolescents who have a chronic or severe acute medical illness are vulnerable to a variety of emotional problems, including depression and anxiety. In both children and adolescents, behavioral problems may be the only apparent evidence for a mood or anxiety disorder. After the initial diagnosis, there may be adjustment difficulties with features of depression and behavioral problems. A lot of fears surface when a person is ill, and particularly for adolescents, the illness may isolate them from their friends, as they begin to feel different. Chronically ill children tend to have reduced socialization with their peers, which in turn can also precipitate or worsen depression. There may be developmental delays across several areas of functioning as a result of the illness, so it is important to seek a mental health evaluation as soon as possible, in an effort to minimize these delays. Therapy can be very useful to address issues of self-esteem and loss of personal control. Group therapy in particular is often very useful for the medically ill, both for adolescents and adults.

80. Why is depression more common in women?

Depression is twice as prevalent in women as in men. This difference, however, does not occur until midpuberty. Childhood depression is more common in boys.

Many theories can explain this difference. One hypothesis as to the higher frequency of depression in women is that hormonal changes occur across the life span. Hormonal and other biological factors have not adequately explained the differences however. It has also been postulated that women may be more likely to report their depressive symptoms, but scientific evidence has not supported this, as studies have demonstrated that men and women are equally likely to report their depressive symptoms.

The symptom profile for men and women tends to be similar, except that women are more apt to report anxious symptoms and physical complaints. In terms of co-morbid conditions, women are more likely to experience concurrent anxiety, and men have behavioral and substance abuse disorders.

Social factors have appeared to have a larger role in the cause of differences between men and women than biological factors. For example, more females than males experience child sexual abuse. Women who have experienced physical or sexual abuse in childhood are at higher risk for developing depression than women who have not been abused. In addition, research has shown that girls experience a higher number of stressful events than boys. Gender roles also may contribute, as some aspects of the feminine role may be more associated with depression. Adolescent girls who are preoccupied with their appearance are vulnerable to depression, and gender inequality in marital relationships also promotes increased rates of depression in women. Females tend to have a more negative self-view than males. Such cognitive thought patterns can increase the likelihood for depression.

81. What are the postpartum blues? Does that mean that I am depressed or will become depressed?

Pregnancy is a time of both physical and emotional changes. It is often expected that women should be happy during their pregnancy, but in fact, because of physical and psychological changes, an increased susceptibility for the onset of a depressive episode exists. Both the pregnancy and the postpartum period are often when a first episode of depression occurs. During the postpartum period, an emotional state called the "blues" commonly occurs. Hormone levels have dropped precipitously. Sleep deprivation occurs, and new psychological factors are at play in response to the woman having a new role as a mother. The blues occur in 50% to 85% of all women postpartum and are characterized by symptoms of depressed mood, tearfulness, mood swings, irritability, and anxiety. These symptoms tend to be self-limited, beginning a few days postpartum and lasting a couple of weeks. If symptoms persist beyond 2 weeks and/or significantly impair functioning, there is a greater likelihood that a major depressive episode is present or will develop.

The postpartum period can be a high-risk time for a depressive episode in vulnerable women. For similar reasons the blues occur, so too can depression. Depression occurs in approximately 10% to 15% of all postpartum women, which approximates the occurrence in the general population. Thus, although hormonal factors are believed to be contributory, they are not strictly causative. Factors associated with an increased risk for postpartum depression are past history of depression, a family history of depression, limited social support and interpersonal conflicts, and negative life events. The majority of women have the onset of symptoms within 6-weeks postpartum. The presence of depression does not signify poor parenting. What is important is to seek treatment right away because untreated depression in the mother can have deleterious effects on the baby's development.

82. I have been diagnosed with postpartum depression. Is my baby at risk?

With recent media coverage of high-profile criminal cases of women who harmed their children while suffering from postpartum illness, the diagnosis of depression in the postpartum period can result in concerns regarding the baby's welfare. The benefit of significant coverage of such tragedies is that it brings into the open and to the attention of clinicians the very real risks of untreated depression in the postpartum period. Although infanticide is in fact a rare outcome of mental illness, the real risks can be subtler. Depression after a birth can result in low self-esteem, reduced confidence in mothering abilities, and decreased attachment and bonding between mother and infant. Depression in the postpartum period is often dismissed as "hormonal" or normal "**baby blues**." In fact, clinical depression is more severe than the baby blues, as it can be associated with suicidal ideation. Untreated depression does have risks other than infanticide which are more likely. A depressed mother will be less in tune to the

Baby blues

common symptoms of sadness and tearfulness that occur in the days after giving birth.

baby's needs, less able to monitor the environment for safety, and less apt to engage in a nonverbal dialogue with the baby. Early attachment is important in a baby's development, as poor attachment confers risks later in life for emotional and behavioral problems. Once diagnosed with depression, however, it is important to understand that with treatment the risks will dissipate. Support from family members or friends can be enlisted to help bridge the gaps in tending to the baby's needs while treatment is initiated. In the majority of instances of postpartum depression, the mother will be able to continue to care for her child while treatment is initiated. Rarely are there circumstances when mother and baby need temporary separation to maintain the baby's safety.

83. I am pregnant and feeling very depressed. Can I take medication?

Treatment of depression during pregnancy can be complicated, as risks to the fetus have to be considered. It has often been difficult for women to obtain medication treatment for depression during pregnancy because of concerns about the effect of medication on the fetus. As no controlled, clinical studies exist that examine medication effects on fetal development, risks versus benefits need to be extrapolated from case reports mainly and based on the individual circumstances for the woman involved. Psychotherapy alone would be the ideal treatment modality but may not be efficacious enough for chronic or moderate to severe depression. Untreated depression can have deleterious effects on the developing fetus itself. Maternal prenatal stress has been associated with lower infant birth weight and gestational age at birth. Animal studies have found that high levels of stress hormones in the maternal blood correlate with behavioral deficits in the offspring. Thus, if you are pregnant and suffering from a severe depression, what medication choices are available? Although no antidepressants have been associated with intrauterine death or major birth defects, few data are available on potential adverse behavioral development in babies exposed to antidepressants *in utero*. One study done on tricyclics did not show any difference in behavioral development. Immediately after birth, however, there have been signs of neonatal withdrawal both from SSRI and TCA exposure, and the FDA has recently issued a warning that SSRIs and venlafaxine can be associated with neonatal distress when taken late in the third trimester. The exact cause of the distress, such as a discontinuation syndrome or serotonin syndrome, is not known. Neonatal withdrawal may be more likely with antidepressants that have a shorter half-life, such as paroxetine, if caused by a discontinuation syndrome. It is possible to avoid a withdrawal situation by tapering off the antidepressant before the anticipated delivery. There are situations in which untreated depression would be expected to be higher risk than use of an antidepressant. If, however, a woman is still concerned about potential harm to the baby, consideration can also be given for ECT, which has no risk on the developing fetus. ECT is a known safe somatic treatment during pregnancy. If psychotic symptoms are present, ECT is most likely the treatment of choice as well so that antipsychotic medication can be avoided.

Of the psychotherapeutic techniques, interpersonal psychotherapy has been shown to be effective for depression in pregnant woman. Other modalities would likely be helpful as well, as described in Question 37. Even if medication is required, psychotherapy is an important part of the treatment.

84. Can I take an antidepressant while I am nursing?

Data regarding use of many medications during breastfeeding are scarce. The FDA gives a category classification for most medications as to whether they are safe during pregnancy or nursing, but this information is not always reliably based on available data. When some medications, such as benzodiazepines, are consumed, they are known to be present in large quantities in breast milk and thus are presumed to be unsafe. In general, all antidepressants are excreted into breast milk. Although differences may exist between antidepressants as to quantities found in breast milk, data are insufficient to make definitive statements about these differences. A case report on paroxetine found no evidence of it in breast milk, thought possibly because of its half-life, but more studies are needed. Both TCAs and SSRIs are generally undetectable in nursing infant blood. Nortriptyline has been the most studied TCA in breastfeeding women. Children exposed to TCAs have been followed through preschool, and no developmental differences have been found compared with children not exposed to TCAs. TCAs, however, are not typically the first-line treatment for depression because of their side effects.

Increasing research has been conducted into the use of SSRIs during breastfeeding because of their relatively safe side-effect profiles. Data are available on the use of fluoxetine, sertraline, paroxetine, citalopram, and fluvoxamine, with sertraline being studied most over the past few years. Although the medication has not usually been detectable in most studies, there have been infrequent reports of detectable serum levels of sertraline, citalopram, and fluoxetine in exposed infants. No adverse developmental or behavioral effects have been detected to date in nursing infants, but no long-term studies exist. Sertraline is generally considered a relatively low risk medication choice, while fluoxetine may have some level of risk associated with it, possibly because of its long half-life. Three cases of colic have been reported in babies with detectable levels of fluoxetine, and some evidence exists for reduced weight gain after birth.

Although for the most part levels of SSRIs are not usually detectable in infant serum, this does not exclude the possibility of the drug having entered the central nervous system. Therefore, until further studies are done, the use of an SSRI needs to be balanced against the risk of untreated depression in a nursing mother, with strong consideration of the benefits of breastfeeding. Four possible choices are as follows:

1. Nurse infant/no medication
2. Nurse infant/take medication
3. Formula feed infant/no medication
4. Formula feed infant/take medication

Clearly, choice number 3 would be the least desirable, as the infant is exposed to maternal depression and not getting the benefits of breast milk. Choice number 1 would offer the infant the benefits of breast milk, but the risk from exposure to maternal depression would likely be greater than the benefits of breastfeeding can offset. Infant exposure to maternal depression for extended periods has been associated with reduced weight gain as well as other complications described in

Question 82. Thus, the decision to balance will likely be between choices 2 and 4. Based on the current literature, the benefits of breastfeeding likely exceed the risk of SSRI exposure, but you will need to go over the choice more thoroughly with your doctor so that you feel comfortable with your decision.

85. After a heart attack 6 months ago, my father has been minimally interested in former activities and is afraid to go anywhere alone. Is this normal?

Depression and heart disease are increasingly being recognized as risk factors for one another. Just as smoking and high cholesterol increase one's odds of developing heart disease, so can the diagnosis of depression. Additionally, the risk of developing depression in the first year after a heart attack is dramatically greater than in the general population, going from 1 in 20 in the general population to 1 in 3 after a heart attack. Depression places a great deal of stress on the body. It can cause levels of stress hormones to rise, leading to increases in cholesterol, blood sugar, and arterial plaques. Depression can affect clotting factors, heart rate and rhythm, and blood pressure, all of which lead to increased chances for heart disease and heart attacks.

Treatment of depression in patients with known heart disease or known family histories of heart disease becomes even more critical for those reasons. Many antidepressants have been studied to determine their safety in cardiac patients after a heart attack and have been found to be as safe as in the general population. Some studies have demonstrated that some antidepressants such as the SSRIs can also directly cause **platelet inhibition** similar to aspirin, thus adding

Platelet inhibition

referring to the inhibition of platelet activity, such as clotting.

another protective measure aside from their antidepressant effects. Currently, studies are underway to demonstrate whether treating depression lowers the rate of recurrent heart attacks, as preliminary studies have suggested. For all of these reasons it is therefore imperative to get your family member into treatment if depression is suspected if he or she has heart disease or after a heart attack.

86. My mother has memory problems. Her doctor diagnosed pseudodementia and prescribed an antidepressant. Is she at risk for Alzheimer's disease?

Pseudodementia is a term that is applied to older patients who initially present to their doctors complaining of memory problems but turn out to have depression. Many similarities exist between patients with dementia and pseudodementia, including apathy, anhedonia, energy disturbance, and sleep and appetite disturbances. In general, however, patients suffering from dementia do not overly complain about their poor memory. In fact, many are completely unaware that they have memory problems. Instead, they often accuse others of "playing with their heads" because they misplaced something and believe that someone has taken it. Patients with pseudodementia often complain bitterly about their loss of memory and frequently refer to themselves as "losing their minds" or "becoming demented." When tests of memory are performed in these patients, however, they demonstrate normal memory. The onset of the memory loss also varies, with patients suffering from pseudodementia having a more rapid onset of memory loss than those suffering from dementia.

Pseudodementia
literally, "false dementia." Depression in older persons can cause cognitive effects that mimic dementia.

Alzheimer's disease
a progressive disease of the brain that is characterized by a gradual loss of cognitive functions such as memory and reasoning.

Why does depression affect memory? Depression often leads to **ruminations**, which is a constant turning over of the same internal thoughts and feelings one can experience when suffering from depression. When locked into ruminations, it is very difficult to attend to the outside world. In addition, when you attempt to concentrate, the energy required for concentration leads to quick fatigue, causing you to be drawn back into your ruminations more easily. When attention and concentration are lost, the ability to input new memories is lost, and therefore, you experience this as a loss of memory. Although pseudodementia can be caused by depression, it can also be caused by prescription medications; even medications as seemingly benign as ibuprofen have been found to cause cognitive problems in the older population.

Ruminations

obsessive thinking over an idea or decision.

Depression is four times more likely to occur in patients over 65 years than in those younger than 65 years. The rates of dementia increase with age as well. Clearly, the rate of depression among patients with dementia is quite high, with approximately 20% to 30% of Alzheimer's patients suffering from depression in addition to their dementia. The link between dementia and pseudodementia was once thought to be weaker than it is considered now, and the diagnosis may actually be a harbinger for the development of dementia later on, although not from direct causation, but rather because the dementia may first present as depression in some cases. In this age group, it is often easy to dismiss symptoms as normal aging or as a normal reaction to the presence of multiple physical problems. This is potentially dangerous because the risk of suicide increases with age, particularly in men. As most patients with pseudodementia respond well to treatment, identification and treatment of pseudodementia is imperative.

87. My mother is in a nursing home and has stopped eating. Her doctor thinks that she is depressed. She never had a mental disorder before. Is this possible?

Depression can occur throughout the lifespan. Even without a history of depression, an older person can become depressed, especially in the context of life stressors. Depression may be masked by medical conditions in older persons. Older adults are less likely to present to their physician with complaints of depression. Physical symptoms of depression may be difficult to differentiate from symptoms of any medical illness the person has or side effects from medication. Sometimes, when depressive symptoms are recognized, it is then falsely assumed that the depression is a normal reaction to changing life circumstances. It is important to recognize depression in older people, as there is a high rate of suicide in this population. Older white men in particular are at the greatest risk for suicide, highlighting the importance of identification and treatment.

Treatment of depression is the same in the older population, although there is higher potential for side effects, and there is more concern for interactions with other medication that may be taken. TCAs and MAOIs have more troublesome side effects for older adults than the SSRIs. SSRIs also need to be chosen carefully because of the potential for harmful drug–drug interactions. Sertraline is commonly prescribed because of its profile in this regard.

In addition to medication management, psychotherapy also should be recommended as part of the treatment. Modification in the therapy may be needed to account for any age-related cognitive changes. A manual-based cognitive therapy treatment has been developed for late-life depression. Interpersonal psychotherapy has also been studied and has been found to be effective for late-life depression.

88. I have low thyroid and take medication. I have been depressed as well. Will my depression get better on the thyroid treatment?

Endocrine disorders such as **hypothyroidism** are associated with psychiatric symptoms, particularly depression and anxiety. Hypothyroidism is a condition that occurs more frequently in women. Symptoms of hypothyroidism that can look like a major depressive episode include the following:

Endocrine disorder
a disorder of the endocrine system, where glands release hormones directly into the blood stream whose actions occur at another site.

Hypothyroidism
decreased or absence of thyroid hormone, causing metabolism to slow, leading to symptoms that can mimic clinical depression.

- Inattentiveness
- Slowing of thought
- Weakness
- Poor memory
- Depressive mood
- Anxiety
- Insomnia
- Psychosis

Typically, physical symptoms are present that would be consistent with a thyroid condition and may include dry skin, thin and dry hair, constipation, stiffness, a coarse voice, facial puffiness, and carpal tunnel symptoms. If a thyroid condition is suspected, blood tests can be done to assess thyroid functioning. If hypothyroidism is present, the treatment for it is typically thyroid supplementation. In most cases, the depression will remit, but some patients will still require treatment for the depression.

Thyroid hormone is often used as an augmenting agent in cases of refractory depression or if only a partial response to an antidepressant is achieved. Thyroid hormone is taken with an antidepressant. No correlation exists between thyroid function and the response to thyroid hormone supplementation, and thus, normal thyroid functioning and laboratory studies do not preclude a trial of thyroid medication if antidepressants are not working.

PART SEVEN

Surviving

What are my rights to refuse hospitalization?

What are my rights to refuse medication and other treatments?

What are my rights to privacy?

More . . .

89. What are my rights to refuse hospitalization?

First, it is important to be aware of the fact that the right to refuse hospitalization varies from state to state. However, most states have fairly similar criteria for involuntary hospitalization or what is also known as civil commitment. Such criteria are that a mental illness is present and that the person is imminently dangerous to self or others. Ways in which the criteria may differ from state to state are primarily on the length of stay allowed before court review and on minor procedural differences. There may also be differences as to whether inclusion of "grave disability" can be added as an additional criterion when deciding to hospitalize an individual involuntarily. Some states do not allow for this. Grave disability means that an individual is so disabled by a mental illness that he or she is in imminent danger. For example, an individual with severe diabetes who has stopped taking insulin because of severe depression would be considered in grave danger of developing a diabetic coma.

It is important to have some historical background in order to understand the basis of one's rights to refuse hospitalization. Involuntary commitment to a psychiatric hospital was first based on the legal term *parens patriae* (Latin for "parent of his country"). Under this doctrine, the state or government, as represented by a physician, acted as the "parent" for the mentally ill individual and could commit him or her to a psychiatric facility merely based on the opinion that the patient was in need of such care. A landmark 1973 case, Lessard vs. Schmidt, in Wisconsin changed this law. Lessard, the plaintiff, was involuntarily committed and argued successfully that her rights were violated because of that commitment. First, she argued that the grounds on which she was committed, the *parens patriae* law, were overly vague by defining a mentally ill individual as one who requires care and treatment for his own welfare or for the welfare of others in the community. Second, she argued that the procedure used to commit her violated her civil rights by denying her due process. The court agreed on both counts, arguing that the patient had all of the rights accorded to a criminal suspect. As a result of this case, *parens patriae* was replaced by the requirement that an individual meet the criteria of being both mentally ill and imminently dangerous in order to be involuntary committed. The courts hoped to decrease the number of admissions to psychiatric hospitals by defining the commitment standards more narrowly, as they considered such action as potentially more damaging than the risks to the individual and community by not committing them.

A second legal ruling occurred in 1976, known as the **Tarasoff** case, after the family of a girl murdered by a man sued for not being warned of the man's threats to murder the girl. The man had told his psychologist of his intentions, and the psychologist notified the police of the man's threats. The police performed their own interview of the man. Based on their interview, no evidence existed that the man was either mentally ill or imminently dangerous, and he was released. The initial court ruling held that both the police and the treating clinicians were responsible, but on appeal, the case against the police was dropped, whereas the clinicians were held to an even greater standard that required of them the duty to protect. With the growing concern

Tarasoff

the name of the family who sued a therapist; consequently, therapists are now required to protect and warn potential victims from violent acts or threats made by patients under their care.

about the increasing liability one accepts for treating individuals with potential for such acts and the fact that there is no science to predict dangerousness, the number of individuals involuntarily committed has skyrocketed, leading to a consequence the courts hoped to avert.

It is important to understand the history behind involuntary commitment to understand rights to refuse hospitalization. Expressing suicidal or homicidal feelings does not automatically mandate immediate hospitalization. Consideration is given to what is said, how it is said, and to whom it is said. The less the clinician knows the patient, the more careful that clinician will be in asking further questions or in referring the patient to an emergency room to be evaluated for hospitalization. Nothing regarding safety is taken lightly under these circumstances, even if one is expressing their feelings in a way that he or she believes is figurative and not literal. It is important to have a strong, trusting relationship with one's treating clinician where all options for treatment can be discussed openly and freely without fear. Under those circumstances, hospitalization may be raised as an option among many others for thorough discussion. The clinician should be able to describe parameters for when hospitalization is considered an absolute necessity. The clinician may ask for outside supports such as family members to be more involved in order to avoid hospitalization. In fact, an adequate support system is one of the single most critical factors in maintaining safety and avoiding hospitalization.

If hospitalized involuntarily, options are available for patients to appeal the commitment. The right to due process and legal representation is maintained. Depending on the state, this may include a court-appointed attorney or a legal advocate. Usually a specific time limit is set by the state within which a patient has a legal right to have a hearing before a judge to request release from the hospital. Hospitals are also required to post a patient's "bill of rights" and to hand them out to every patient. Even when involuntarily committed, patients continue to have the right to refuse treatment and cannot be medicated without consent unless a clear and immediate danger toward self or others is evident. This is typically a one-time dose of a short-acting medication to help calm one and is also known legally as a chemical restraint. Physical restraint or seclusion may also be applied to prevent a patient from harming one's self or others. Specific requirements are mandated by the federal government regarding the application of such restraints, including appropriate monitoring and documentation of restraint usage, and specific time limits within which re-evaluation by a physician is required.

90. What are my rights to refuse medication and other treatments?

Unlike involuntary hospitalization where issues of safety trump autonomy, the right to refuse treatment continues to be sacrosanct (except as noted in Question 89 regarding the use of "chemical restraints"). In general, patients have the absolute right to refuse medical or psychiatric treatment of any kind, short of emergency hospitalization for issues of safety. The clinician must obtain **informed consent** before prescribing any treatment. Informed consent is a legal and ethical doctrine fundamental to modern medicine. The

Informed consent
the premise that patients have a right to determine what happens to their body.

process of obtaining informed consent includes the following elements:

- Assessment of the patient's capacity to make medical decisions
- Absence of coercion of the patient
- Fully informing the patient of his or her diagnosis and prognosis, risks versus benefits of the treatment offered, risks versus benefits of alternative treatments, and risks versus benefits of receiving no treatment

There are few but notable exceptions to informed consent. These exceptions include emergencies, therapeutic privilege, therapeutic waiver, and implied consent. In many emergency situations, the patient is unconscious and in need of life-saving treatment. Informed consent is assumed or obtained to the best of the clinician's ability. When clinicians assume therapeutic privilege, they are withholding information from the patient because they believe that informing the patient will cause more harm then good. Occasionally patients will request not to be informed. In other words, they waive their right to be informed. Such a waiver is not advisable. One should enlist the aid of a family member to make decisions when one wants to remove oneself from the decision. Finally, implied consent occurs when one offers one's arm to have blood drawn or their blood pressure checked.

When refusing medication or treatment, it is important to be informed of and understand the potential consequences of refusing. Understanding the consequences requires one to have the capacity to refuse treatment. The capacity to refuse treatment requires four elements:

- The ability to express a choice
- The ability to understand the treatment options and their consequences
- The ability to appreciate the information as it applies to one's specific situation
- The ability to reason with the information

All four elements must be met for a patient to have the capacity to decide on medical or psychiatric treatment. Obviously, most of these elements are generally understood between the patient and the clinician in most treatment decisions. These become important to sort out more clearly when someone is in a life-threatening situation and is refusing a life-saving treatment. Under those circumstances, a physician may call in a psychiatrist to evaluate one's capacity to refuse treatment, and if one lacks such capacity, he or she may recommend an emergency conservatorship in order to help make such decisions. Usually, a family member is appointed the conservator under those circumstances.

There are fewer, although real, life-threatening psychiatric conditions even after someone has been hospitalized. The most obvious is when a patient remains out of control behaviorally and requires a chemical restraint. Less obvious is a patient so severely depressed that he or she is no longer eating or drinking and is refusing all treatment. Under these circumstances, in most states, a conservatorship hearing will only allow for medical treatments to maintain the person's life but will not allow for the administration of psychiatric treatment if that individual continues to refuse that form of care. In fact, conservators generally only have the right to make decisions about medical care, housing, and finances. Conservators cannot sign someone into a psychiatric hospital, and they cannot agree to have a person forcibly medicated. Instead, a second hearing must occur, during which independent psychiatrists review the case and report their findings to the court. Only then will a judge determine whether a person can receive psychiatric care against his or her will in the form of medication or some other therapy. This procedure typically occurs after a patient is hospitalized but continues to refuse medication. Under such circumstances, the hospital pursues this course of action because it is believed that the patient's health and well-being depend on treatment.

As an outpatient, it is important to understand and weigh the treatment options to the best of one's ability and to enlist outside support from other informative sources if needed. The right to refuse medication as an outpatient is respected the vast majority of the time. In fact, few states allow for involuntary outpatient treatment. This is changing, however, in very specific and limited circumstances. Recent high-profile cases in various states where noncompliant mentally ill patients have injured or killed someone have prompted new involuntary outpatient treatment laws. However, the requirements imposed on caregivers for making their case for involuntary treatment are exceedingly stringent and require regular court review.

91. What are my rights to privacy?

The issue of confidentiality has become one of the hottest issues in medicine in the past few years with the introduction of the new federal laws encompassed under the acronym HIPAA (Health Insurance Portability and Accountability Act). The field of medicine has always regarded confidentiality as one of its highest ethical principles. Psychiatry has put even greater restrictions on confidentiality given the highly sensitive nature of the issues patients discuss. As a result, no information is released to anyone without a written authorization by the patient allowing for such release. A written authorization for release of general medical records is not enough. The patient must knowingly and specifically request psychiatric and/or drug and alcohol information to be released before it can be. Every effort is made to protect a patient's right to privacy.

However, exceptions exist to that right, and it behooves everyone to know what those exceptions are. First, confidentiality does not apply when a patient is considered to be a threat to others, unless hospitalized. Second, confidentiality does not apply when the law requires mandatory reporting. This includes communicable diseases, child or elder abuse, impaired driving, and any other requirement in a particular jurisdiction. Third, depending on the state, court-ordered or subpoenaed records can be released without the patient's written authorization. However, a good clinician will usually notify the patient and attempt to obtain written authorization before honoring the court's request. Certain states (such as Connecticut) have laws that supercede the Federal HIPAA laws on "protected" records subpoenaed by the court. Most states still require a HIPAA authorization for release to the court be signed by the patient. If a signed patient authorization cannot be obtained, appropriate steps should be taken under state law by the clinician to object to the subpoena. These actions usually involve engaging an attorney to file such motions in the state court system.

Fourth, hospitals and offices may release minimally necessary healthcare information without the patient's written permission for the purposes of treatment, payment, or operations (such as quality control, peer review, and teaching). This is encompassed under the HIPAA rules (discussed later here).

The most important factor to bear in mind when a clinician releases psychiatric information about a patient to another person without that patient's consent is the concept of "duty to third parties." Most lawyers would prefer to defend a breach of confidentiality case than a wrongful death case. Clinician's understand this very well and in emergency situations may feel obligated to violate a patient's autonomy and confidentiality in order to protect him or her and the community from some greater harm. This is especially true if the patient is being evaluated in an emergency room. In those instances, clinicians will generally not feel comfortable discharging a patient before obtaining outside sources of information, and refusing to allow such contact will only delay discharge and probably ensure hospitalization under an involuntary commitment. A good clinician, however, will always inform the patient of his or her decisions and whom they are contacting.

The initial impetus behind HIPAA was to extend the ability of people to maintain their healthcare insurance after termination of employment and decrease the exclusions for pre-existing conditions. HIPAA was also an attempt by the government to provide further controls over fraud and abuse of the Medicare system as well as standardize the electronic claims system between providers and third-party vendors. However, to most people, HIPAA has become synonymous with privacy because one of the first orders of business when one enters a doctor's office today is to receive a notice of privacy practice and sign that one received such notice. The notice of privacy practice outlines the rights of the patient regarding privacy and the provider's duty to protect the health information generated within the office or entity, describing the various ways in which one's healthcare information can be shared without requiring written permission unless the person objects to any such release in writing beforehand as outlined earlier. Again, the notice also outlines the release of healthcare information as mandated by law as pointed out previously here. Additionally, it specifically mentions that psychiatric and drug and alcohol information are specially protected, although limited amounts of information on these diagnoses may be shared for the purposes of treatment, payment, or operations. The notice specifically states that unless provided with a written request it is assumed that information such as appointments can be shared via phone, mail, or with family members, etc. Finally, patients have the right to view and amend their healthcare information by submitting a written request. This can be denied under specific circumstances outlined in the notice, but the patient has a right to know the reasons and may appeal such denials.

Generally, when one first enters a doctor's office and begins filling out a myriad of forms, one form will be to authorize release of information for purposes of treatment, payment, and operations. With respect to payment, one's health insurance company requires medical information for the purposes of payment because it wants to know what it is paying for. The term that insurance companies use to authorize payment is "medical necessity," meaning that they want proof that the bill sent to them for a particular service was medically necessary and therefore deserving of payment. This also means that the clinician must send the insurer the diagnosis and the treatment rendered in order to demonstrate medical necessity, which may include copies of the clinician's documentation. If a patient refuses to allow the release of such information, either the clinician may refuse to see or treat the patient, or if seen, the patient will be responsible for the bill. Again, it was the purpose of HIPAA to provide the patient with the right to make an informed decision on his or her health information privacy.

92. *Is it necessary to involve my family in my treatment?*

Anne's comment:

When one family member is experiencing depression, the entire family is affected. In our situation, when both of our adolescent children were in crisis with their bipolar disorders, the stress caused my spouse to begin to recede into a depression, and I had to struggle to maintain a healthy perspective with so many ill family members to care for. Being involved in each family member's individual therapy and having regular family therapy sessions were essential to keeping a family in crisis together.

Although the decision about the level of involvement of a family member in the evaluation and treatment of depression is generally up to you, your clinician may request (and in certain circumstances insist) that an involved family member be brought in as part of the evaluation process. Depression typically affects a person's cognitive abilities and can be so severe that the ability to make decisions becomes impaired. The involvement of a family member helps to clarify symptoms, relationship and work difficulties, as well as family history. The involved family member may have certain insights as to recent stressors that triggered the onset of the depressive episode. Most importantly, your family member can be an important supportive figure during the initial phase of treatment and the recovery process. Sometimes depressed persons only seek treatment at the insistence of their loved ones. Because of effects on motivation, self-esteem, and feelings of self-sufficiency, a depressed person may not engage fully in the treatment process. The person may need reminders to take his or her medication and keep appointments. Even more important, if you are having suicidal thinking, an involved family member may be an important factor that your clinician uses in determining your ability to be safe. A family member can monitor for suicidal behaviors. If a person is alone and without any support network, he or she is at higher risk for complications of depression, including suicide. Thus, a clinician may insist a family member be involved in the treatment if it is believed a person's personal safety is at risk.

93. I am worried about my employer finding out about my treatment.

Many employers are actually paying the medical bills through contracts established with health insurance companies. As a result, they often feel entitled to know what they are paying for. Additionally, if you take time off work for depression you may be concerned about what will be released to your employer to justify the time off. Finally, in many job application forms, the issue of a mental disability comes up as part of the application process. All of these issues may lead to concern that your employer will gain knowledge of your illness and that negative consequences will result from such knowledge. Although all of these issues are of concern, paying the bill does not give an employer the right to specific information beyond the minimum amount necessary. They are on a "need to know" basis. They have no right to know your diagnosis, whether it is medical or psychiatric, for either payment or time away from work. An employer may request information on whether the illness will impact on job performance in any way in order to know whether you should remain out of work or return with a change or reduction in workload. Finally, any application for employment should ask only if you are suffering from a mental disability that would impair your ability to perform your job. Depression is a treatable mental illness and is *not* in and of itself a disability. The obvious answer to such a question then is "no." The vast majority of people treated for depression can expect a full recovery to their previous functional capacity. You do not need to disclose to a potential employer that you have been treated or that you continue to receive treatment for depression.

94. Will I get depressed again after I have recovered?

Many people who have a major depressive episode go for many years without another episode of depression. Remission is defined as the absence of or presence of only minimal symptoms with normal functionality. Once remission has lasted for more than 6 months, it is considered recovery. If full recovery has been achieved, a subsequent episode of depression is considered a recurrence. The risk of recurrence drops with increasing time since the index episode. The risk for recurrence is highest within the first year after recovery. The risk for recurrence is also affected by the number of episodes of depression that you have had. The greater the number of episodes that you have had, the greater is your risk for becoming depressed again. You can modify your risk for recurrence using the methods described previously in Question 32.

Response to a treatment is defined as a significant improvement of symptoms, but without being completely free of symptoms. Another term for this is **partial remission**. It is important to remember that although many effective treatments for depression are available, response and recovery may not occur with the first treatment intervention. Less than half of depressed persons achieve remission with a trial of a single antidepressant. Keeping this in mind, it is very possible that another medication will need to be tried or that your physician will recommend other strategies. Current research efforts are geared toward facilitating complete remission of depression in most persons. The potential consequences of failing to achieve remission include an increased risk for relapse and later treatment resistance, impaired work functioning, and an increased cost of healthcare.

Partial remission

symptoms of an illness have resolved by 50%.

95. What can I do if I have failed several forms of medication and therapy?

Anne's comment:

Both my spouse and my son have been fortunate in responding well to medication. My daughter's experience has been much more difficult. It took patience and perseverance on her part and diligence on the part of her doctor to achieve a mix of medications that finally stabilized the illness. It is important to resist feelings of hopelessness during this period of discovery.

Unfortunately, situations come about when depression does not respond to conventional treatments available. This can be frustrating and certainly contributes to the morbidity of depression. If you have been with the same clinician, sometimes it can be helpful to obtain a consultation by another clinician who will examine the treatment history and perhaps make some other suggestions. Sometimes lack of response to treatment is due to inadequate dosing or duration of medication trials or due to a missed diagnosis. Co-morbid conditions can make a depressive illness more refractory to treatment. Conditions that may co-occur with depression include anxiety disorders (panic disorder, generalized anxiety disorder, obsessive–compulsive disorder, social anxiety disorder), posttraumatic stress disorder (also an anxiety condition), attention deficit disorder, and substance abuse disorders. Further evaluation and treatment of other conditions may be necessary. Substance abuse treatment, for example, may need to be obtained in order for the depression to be adequately treated. Sometimes a refractory depression is a missed bipolar depression, which may require the use of additional medications. Psychiatrists use guidelines in the treatment of refractory depression. Oftentimes, older antidepressants such as TCAs or MAOIs have yet to be tried, and also ECT may need consideration. Although all psychiatrists are trained in psychopharmacologic treatments, some individuals have a specific expertise in the field of psychopharmacology for depression. These individuals are typically associated with an academic institution. In addition, research protocols are usually being conducted in association with academic institutions investigating newer medications. Participation in a research protocol usually involves a comprehensive evaluation during which other diagnostic possibilities are investigated as well.

96. What is the risk of suicide when someone is diagnosed with depression?

The majority of depressed persons do not attempt suicide, but the majority of suicide attempters have depression. Suicide is the most significant risk of untreated depression. Typically, suicide is not a sudden thought and action; rather, it undergoes development over time. There may initially be only fleeting thoughts of death or wishes of dying. These thoughts can progress to fantasies of methods of killing oneself and later to stages of planning actual self-harm. The time frame of this progression can take as long as weeks to months to as little as within minutes. Someone with poor impulse control may be more apt to attempt suicide within the shorter time period. Anyone with plans to kill oneself or who has made an attempt requires emergency psychiatric evaluation. In some situations, a family member finds out that someone has tried to kill himself or herself but does not take him or her to an emergency room because he or she assures the family member that it was a mistake and that he or she will be okay. It is best, however, if a professional evaluates the situation to determine the most appropriate course of action.

Suicide is the most serious risk of depression. Clinicians assess suicide risk based on many factors, including the patient's current mental status, personal history, family history, use of substances, and more. As stated, suicidal thinking tends to fall on a continuum from morbid thoughts of death to passive thoughts of wishing to be dead to an actual plan to carry out the suicide, a continuum that is assessed by the clinician. Clinicians will ask direct questions about suicidal thoughts. Direct questions do not put ideas in a person's mind; rather, they invite the individual to speak openly about the issue. Most patients want help and want to let someone know how they are feeling. Also in this light, if you have reason to believe a family member is contemplating suicide, it is best to speak openly and frankly about your concerns. Doing so will not put new thoughts of suicide into the person's mind; instead, it will give an opportunity to help him or her get the treatment that may be needed.

97. A family member committed suicide. I feel guilty that I missed something.

Anne's comment:

Sadly, we experienced the loss of my husband's mother to suicide when our children were very young. That traumatic event has made us vigilant in getting professional help for us and for our children when the need arises. Although there is sometimes a possibility that a patient will commit suicide despite the best care and treatment, it is helpful to focus on the greater likelihood that treatment will prevent such a traumatic end to a loved one's suffering and will restore the depressed person to a state of well-being.

Suicide is the single most tragic outcome of patients suffering from mental illness. No matter how prepared someone thinks he or she is that a family member may eventually commit suicide because of his or her pain and suffering, it always feels unexpected and comes as a complete surprise. When it happens, everyone, including family, friends, and caregivers, feels shocked. Some are completely devastated with guilt about the loss. Small, seemingly insignificant events leading up to the person's death, appearing at the time to be normal, take on a new and painful meaning in retrospect. These events evolve into clear signs of the person's commitment to the inevitable last act, thus heightening the feelings of guilt. A sense of having let the person down, of saying the wrong thing, or of not being there when he or she needed you most may be present. When looked at in retrospect, everyone asks himself or herself, "How could I have missed that?" These are normal feelings.

An exact science of predicting suicide is not presently established and probably never will be established. Some people live their lives with chronic suicidal ideation and never act on their thoughts. Some people engage in countless acts of cutting and overdosing without any significant physical harm to themselves. Alternatively, other people have never thought of suicide their entire lives until the moment that they commit suicide. Despite the advances psychiatry has made in assessing and treating mental illness, it is only one of many risk factors that contribute to suicide. Epidemiologists develop risk factors by looking at population aggregates of people who attempt or complete suicide and establishing the frequency that various factors correlate with suicide; however, correlation does not mean causation. Although risk factors can help to assess someone who is at risk for suicide, they play little role in helping to predict whether and when a person at risk will attempt or complete suicide. As a result, psychiatry is an inexact science at best, and the ability to predict suicide is worse than forecasting the weather. One can never underestimate the power of free will. Although guilt is a feeling one cannot control and is often a normal expected response under such circumstances, one is rarely guilty for another's actions.

98. My psychiatrist tells me he has a "duty to warn" if I become threatening. What does that mean?

"Duty to warn" is the direct result of a famous 1974 legal case known as Tarasoff, updated to "duty to protect" after an appeal in 1976. The Tarasoff case, as described in Question 89, is named after the family of a girl, murdered by a man, who sued because the girl was not warned of the man's threats to murder her. "Duty to warn" refers to a legal and ethical obligation that healthcare providers have to third parties who are in danger because of threats made by their patients while under their care. This duty trumps all rights to confidentiality with respect to your privacy when confiding in a therapist or physician. In many ways, it is legally similar to providers' obligation to notify the state child abuse agency if they have a suspicion of abuse. It is one of the HIPAA privacy exceptions outlined in the Notice of Privacy Acts in order "to avert serious threat to health or safety."

This duty to warn does not apply to a patient's expression of suicidal thoughts, although families of patients who committed suicide have sued clinicians for such rights because of a clinician's failure to notify them. In a case on the subject known as Bellah v. Greeson

(1978) the court ruled against the idea of a Tarasoff-like warning to the patient's family, citing the greater obligation to protect confidentiality in order to encourage patients to seek treatment they would otherwise refuse if they knew their family would be notified. Legal experts and clinicians have, however, continued to suggest and recommend the notification of family as a serious option when a patient presents as a risk to himself or herself. Usually, under those circumstances, if a clinician believes a patient is imminently suicidal, that clinician has the higher duty to protect his or her patient, which essentially obligates the clinician to hospitalize the patient either voluntarily or involuntarily.

99. What is NAMI? How can they help?

NAMI, an acronym for the National Alliance for the Mentally Ill, is an advocacy group that is made up predominantly of family members of patients and patients themselves who are suffering from mental illness. As its mission statement reports, "NAMI is dedicated to the eradication of mental illnesses and to the improvement of the quality of life of all those whose lives are affected by these diseases." From its inception in 1979, NAMI has worked very hard to advocate for the mentally ill in order to achieve equitable services and treatment for more than 15 million patients and their families in need. It is an all-volunteer organization with more than a thousand local chapters in all 50 states that provide education to consumers and the community, lobby for increased research, and provide advocacy for health insurance, housing, rehabilitation, and jobs for those struggling with mental illness. As each community has unique characteristics and needs, each chapter serves to meet these needs on an individual community basis. Their website, *www.nami.org*, can provide further information and resources for those interested in becoming involved in their local chapters.

100. Where can I find out more information about depression?

It is not possible to discuss all possible aspects of depression in one small volume. Appendix A contains organizations, hotline numbers, and websites that can be useful to patients with depression and their families.

Appendix A

Organizations

American Foundation for Suicide Prevention
120 Wall Street, 22nd Floor
New York, NY 10005
(888) 333-AFSP
www.afsp.org

Depression and Bipolar Support Alliance
730 N. Franklin Street, Suite 501
Chicago, IL 60610-7224
(800) 826-3632
www.dbsalliance.org

Depression and Related Affective Disorders Association
2330 West Joppa Rd.
Suite 100
Lutherville, MD 21093
(410) 583-2919
www.drada.org

Families for Depression Awareness
300 Fifth Avenue
Waltham, MA 02451
(781) 890-0220
www.familyaware.org

National Alliance for the Mentally Ill
Colonial Place Three
2107 Wilson Blvd., Suite 300
Arlington, VA 22201-3042
(703) 524-7600
www.nami.org

National Institute of Mental Health
Office of Communications
6001 Executive Boulevard, Room 8184, MSC 9663
Bethesda, MD 20892-9663
(301) 443-4513
www.nimh.nih.gov

National Mental Health Association
2001 N. Beauregard Street, 12th Floor
Alexandria, VA 22311
(800) 969-NMHA
www.nmha.org

Food and Drug Administration
5600 Fishers Lane
Rockville, Maryland 20857
(888) INFO-FDA
www.fda.gov

Hotline Numbers

National Adolescent Suicide Hotline
(800) 621-4000

National Drug and Alcohol Treatment Hotline
(800) 662-HELP

National Suicide Prevention Lifeline
(800) 273-TALK

National Youth Crisis Hotline
(800) HIT-HOME

Websites

www.aabt.org
Association for Advancement of Behavior Therapy website with link to find a therapist

www.aacap.org
American Academy of Child and Adolescent Psychiatry website with resources for patients and their families

www.aboutourkids.org
NYU Child Study Center website on child mental health

www.academyofct.org
The Academy of Cognitive Therapy website with links for consumer information and finding a certified cognitive therapist

www.apahelpcenter.org
American Psychological Association website with articles and information for consumers

www.bazelon.org
Bazelon Center for Mental Health Law website with information pertaining to their work in national legal advocacy for the mentally ill

www.depressioncenter.net
An interactive website with online support available

www.dr-bob.org
Psychopharmacology tips

www.healthfinder.gov
U.S. Department of Health and Human Service sponsored site that connects to resources on the web pertaining to health related information.

www.human-nature.com
Clearing house for all aspects of human behavior

www.mentalhealth.org
U.S. Department of Health and Human Service website for mental health information

www.nacbt.org
National Association of Cognitive-Behavioral Therapists website with information for consumers and link to find a certified cognitive-behavioral therapist

www.naswdc.org/resources
National Association of Social Workers website with listing of social workers meeting national standards

www.psych.org/public_info/
American Psychiatric Association website with section on public information for patients

www.webmd.org
Website providing medical and health and wellness information

Appendix B

Medication generic (Trade name)	Typical Dosing Range[1]	Max Dosage Recommended[2]	Available Form	Cost/month[3]
SSRIs				
fluoxetine (Prozac)	20–60 mg	80 mg	tab, cap, liquid	$80–$250
sertraline (Zoloft)	50–200 mg	200 mg	tab, liquid	$80–$200
paroxetine (Paxil, CR)	20–75 mg	60 or 75 (CR) mg	tab, liquid	$100–$200
fluvoxamine (Luvox)	100–300 mg	300 mg	tab	$80–$240
citalopram (Celexa)	20–60 mg	60 mg	tab, liquid	$80–$160
escitalopram (Lexapro)	10–20 mg	20 mg	tab, liquid	$70–$110
TCAs				
clomipramine (Anfranil)	100–250 mg	250 mg	cap	$60–$150
amitriptyline (Elavil)	150–300 mg	300 mg	tab	$35–$100
doxepin (Sinequan)	150–300 mg	300 mg	cap, liquid	$35–$80
trimipramine (Surmontil)	150–300 mg	300 mg	cap	$80–$280
amoxepine (Asendin)	200–400 mg	600 mg	tab	$100–$200
protriptyline (Vivactil)	15–60 mg	60 mg	tab	$70–$280
desipramine (Norpramin)	150–300 mg	300 mg	tab	$65–$135
nortriptyline (Pamelor)	75–150 mg	150 mg	cap, liquid	$65–$130
imipramine (Tofranil)	150–300 mg	300 mg	tab	$60–$120
maprotiline (Ludiomil)	75–225 mg	225 mg	tab	$30–$85

(continued)

Medication generic (Trade name)	Typical Dosing Range[1]	Max Dosage Recommended[2]	Available Form	Cost/month[3]
MAOIs				
phenelzine (Nardil)	45–90 mg	90 mg	tab	$50–$100
tranylcypromine (Parnate)	30–60 mg	60 mg	tab	$75–$150
Others				
trazodone (Desyrel)	150–600 mg	600 mg	tab	$45–$180
venlafaxine (Effexor, XR)	75–375 mg	375 or 225 (XR) mg	tab, cap	$60–$260
mirtazapine (Remeron)	15–45 mg	45 mg	tab	$80–$125
nefazodone (Serzone)	300–600 mg	600 mg	tab	$75–$150
bupropion (Wellbutrin, SR, LA)	300–450 mg	450 or 400 (SR) mg	tab	$85–$220
duloxetine (Cymbalta)	20-60 mg	60 mg	cap	$95–$200

[1]Average range for effective dose, but starting dose may be lower. Also, target doses may be reduced in children and older persons.

[2]Maximum dosage recommended is the manufacturer guideline that is FDA approved. In clinical practice, dosing may be higher.

[3]Costs are approximate only and based on generics if available with a range approximated from the cost of a 30-day supply of various doses within the typical dosing range listed for depression per day. While pills of various strengths are typically similar in cost, the need for half doses or 2 or more pills will result in greater cost, for example.

Glossary

Addiction: continued use of a mood-altering substance despite physical, psychological, or social harm. It is characterized by a lack of control in the amount and frequency of use, cravings, continued use in the presence of adverse effects, denial of negative consequences, and a tendency to abuse other mood-altering substances.

Adoption study: a scientific study designed to control for genetic relatedness and environmental influences by comparing siblings adopted into different families.

Akathisia: a subjective sense of inner restlessness resulting in the need to keep moving. Objectively, restless movements or pacing may be signs of akathisia.

Algorithm: a sequence of steps to follow when approaching a particular problem.

Alternative treatment: a treatment for a medical condition that has not undergone scientific studies to demonstrate its efficacy.

Alzheimer's disease: a progressive disease of the brain that is characterized by a gradual loss of cognitive functions such as memory and reasoning. Personality and behavioral changes can accompany the disease as it progresses.

Anticonvulsant: a drug that controls or prevents seizures. Anticonvulsants often are used in psychiatric practice to treat mania, mood instability, or other mental conditions.

Antidepressant: a drug specifically marketed for and capable of relieving the symptoms of clinical depression. It is often used to treat conditions other than depression.

Antipsychotic: a drug that treats psychotic symptoms, such as hallucinations, delusions, and thought disorders. Antipsychotics can be used to treat certain mood disorders as well.

Anxiolytic: a substance that relieves subjective and objective symptoms of anxiety.

Attachment: the psychological connection between a child and his or her caretaker. Infants develop attachment behaviors within the first month. Deficits in early attachments can result in problems in later relationships in life.

Atypical antipsychotic: a second-generation antipsychotic with a profile of targeted brain receptors that differs from the older antipsychotics, which have fewer neurologic side effects and also have mood-stabilizing effects.

Augmentation: in pharmacotherapy, a strategy of using a second medication to enhance the positive effects of an existing medication in the regimen.

Automatic thoughts: thoughts that occur spontaneously whenever a specific, common event occurs in one's life and that are often associated with depression.

Axon: a single fiber of a nerve cell through which a message is sent via an electrical impulse to a receiving neuron. Each nerve cell has one axon.

Baby blues: common symptoms of sadness and tearfulness that occur in the days after giving birth that are thought to be the result of hormonal changes associated with the birth event.

Basal ganglia: a region of the brain consisting of three groups of nerve cells (called the caudate nucleus, putamen, and the globus pallidus) that are collectively responsible for control of movement. Abnormalities in the basal ganglia can result in involuntary movement disorders.

Benzodiazepine: a drug that is part of a class of medication with sedative and anxiolytic effects. Drugs in this class share a common chemical structure and mechanism of action.

Bereavement: the period of time spent in mourning for the death of a loved one.

Biogenic amines: a group of compounds in the nervous system that participate in the regulation of brain activity, including dopamine, serotonin, and norepinephrine.

Biopsychosocial: a model used to describe the possible origins of risk factors for the development of various mental illnesses, incorporating the biological, psychological, and societal factors for a given individual.

Bipolar depression: an episode of depression that occurs in the course of bipolar disorder.

Bipolar disorder: a mental illness defined by episodes of mania or hypomania, classically alternating with episodes of depression. However, the condition can take various forms, such as repeated episodes of mania only or a lack of alternating episodes.

Brainstem: the anatomical part of the brain that connects the brain cortex to the spinal cord. It contains the major centers that regulate what are known collectively as "vegetative functions," that is, sleep, appetite, blood pressure, temperature, and respiration.

Cardiac toxicity: damage that occurs to the heart or coronary arteries as a result of medication side effects.

Catastrophic thinking: a type of automatic thought during which the individual quickly assumes the worst outcome for a given situation.

Central nervous system: nerve cells and their support cells in the brain and spinal cord.

Cerebral cortex: the outer portion of the brain, which is comprised of gray matter and made up of numerous folds that greatly increase the surface area of the brain. Advanced motor function, social abilities, language, and problem solving are coordinated in this area of the brain.

Chemical imbalance: a common vernacular for what is thought to be occurring in the brain in patients suffering from mental illness.

Classical conditioning: a type of learning that results when a conditioned and an unconditioned stimulus is associated, resulting in a similar response to both stimuli (see Pavlovian).

Cognitive behavioral therapy: a combination of cognitive and behavioral approaches in psychotherapy, during which the therapist focuses on automatic thoughts and behavior of a self-defeating quality in order to make one more conscious of them and replace them with more positive thoughts and behaviors.

Co-morbid: the presence of two or more mental disorders, such as depression and anxiety.

Compliance: extent that behavior follows medical advice, such as by taking prescribed treatments. Compliance can refer to medications as well as to appointments and psychotherapy sessions.

Concordance: in genetics, a similarity in a twin pair with respect to presence or absence of illness.

Constitution: referring to a person's biopsychological make-up, that is, the personality and the traits.

Contingency contracting: a behavioral therapy technique that utilizes reinforcers or rewards to modify behaviors.

Countertransferance: the attitudes, opinions, and behaviors that a therapist attributes to his or her patient, not based on the true nature of the patient but rather the biased nature of the therapist because the patient reminds the therapist of his or her own past relationships.

Dependence: the body's reliance on a drug to function normally. Physical dependence results in withdrawal when the drug is stopped suddenly. Dependence should be contrasted to addiction.

Depression: a medical condition associated with changes in thoughts, moods, and behaviors.

Discontinuation syndrome: physical symptoms that occur when a drug is suddenly stopped.

Diurnal variation: a variation in mood that occurs within a day. Patients with clinical depression commonly experience a diurnal variation in mood such that it is worse after awakening but improves as the day progresses.

Double depression: the co-occurrence of a major depressive episode with dysthymic disorder.

Dynamic: referring to a type of therapy that focuses on one's interpersonal relationships, developmental experiences, and the transference relationship with his or her therapist. It is also known as insight-oriented.

Dysthymic: the presence of chronic, mild depressive symptoms.

ECT: electroconvulsive or shock therapy.

Efficacy: the capacity to produce a desired effect, such as the performance of a drug or therapy in relieving symptoms of depression, such as feeling down, trouble concentrating, etc.

Electrochemically: the mechanism by which signals are transmitted neurologically. Brain chemicals, or neurotransmitters, alter the electrical conductivity of nerve tissue, causing a signal to be transmitted or sent.

Emotional memory: a memory evoked by a sensory experience.

Endocrine disorder: a disorder of the endocrine system. Endocrine glands release chemicals (also known as hormones) directly into the blood stream whose actions occur at another site. Endocrine glands include the thyroid, ovaries and testes, adrenals, and pancreas.

Enzyme: a protein made in the body that serves to break down or create other molecules. Enzymes serve as catalysts to biochemical reactions in the body.

Extrapyramidal: the parts of the brain that are responsible for static motor control. The basal ganglia are part of this system. Deficits in this system result in involuntary movement disorders. Antipsychotic medications affect these areas leading to extrapyramidal side effects, which include muscle spasms (dystonias), tremors, shuffling gait, restlessness (akathisia), and tardive dyskinesias.

Fight or flight: a reaction in the body that occurs in response to an immediate threat. Adrenaline is released, which allows for rapid energy to run (flight) or to face the threat (fight).

First-degree relative: immediate biologically related family member, such as biological parents or full siblings.

Flooding: a behavioral therapy technique that involves exposure to the maximal level of anxiety as quickly as possible.

Free association: the mental process of saying aloud whatever comes to mind, suppressing the natural tendency to censor or filter thoughts. This is a technique used in psychoanalysis and in psychodynamic psychotherapy.

Functional: generally referring to a symptom or condition that has no clearly defined physiological or anatomical cause.

Gene: DNA sequence that codes for a specific protein or that regulates other genes. Genes are heritable.

Graded exposure: a psychotherapeutic technique that utilizes gradual exposure through a hierarchy of anxiety-provoking situations. This may begin with imagery techniques first and then progress with limited exposure in time and intensity before full exposure occurs.

Grandiosity: the tendency to consider the self or one's ideas better or more superior to what is reality.

Gray matter: the part of the brain that contains the nerve cell bodies, including the cell nucleus and its metabolic machinery as opposed to the axons, which are essentially the "transmission wires" of the nerve cell. The cerebral cortex contains gray matter.

Half-life: the time it takes for half of the blood concentration of a medication to be eliminated from the body. Half-life determines as well the time to equilibrium of a drug in the blood and determines the frequency of dosing to achieve that equilibrium.

Hormonal: referring to the chemicals that are secreted by the endocrine glands and act throughout the body.

Hyperarousal: a heightened state of alertness to external and internal stimuli, often resulting in sleep disturbance, problems concentrating, hypervigilance, and exaggerated startle response. This is typically seen in posttraumatic conditions.

Hypersomnia: an inability to stay awake. Oversleeping.

Hypomanic: a milder form of mania with the same symptoms but of lesser intensity.

Hypothyroidism: decreased or absence of thyroid hormone, which is secreted by an endocrine gland near the throat and has wide metabolic effects. When thyroid hormone is low, metabolism can slow leading to symptoms that can mimic clinical depression.

Insight-oriented: see dynamic. A form of psychotherapy that focuses on one's developmental history, interpersonal relationships with one's family of origin, and current relationships with friends, spouses, and others. Usually, such relationships are explored through the development of a transference relationship with one's therapist.

Informed consent: the premise that patients have a right to determine what happens to their body and as such agreement to a treatment requires receipt of information, competence to make the decision, and agreeability for the treatment.

Interpersonal therapy: a form of therapy. Unlike insight-oriented or dynamic therapy that focuses on developmental relationships, interpersonal therapy focuses strictly on current relationships and conflicts within them.

Insomnia: the inability to fall asleep, middle of the night awakening, or early morning awakening.

Learned helplessness: a behavioral pattern that occurs after repeated exposure to noxious stimuli that is characterized by withdrawal, passivity, and reduced activity level.

Limbic system: the part of the brain thought to be related to feeding, mating, and most importantly to emotion and memory of emotional events. Brain regions within this system include the hypothalamus, hippocampus, amygdala, and cingulate gyrus, as well as portions of the basal ganglia.

Malignant hypertension: elevated blood pressure that is acute and rapidly progressive with severe symptoms, including headache.

Mania: a condition characterized by elevation of mood (extreme euphoria or irritability) associated with racing thoughts, decreased need for sleep, hyperactivity, and poor impulse control. One episode of mania (in the absence of an ingested substance) is needed to diagnose bipolar disorder.

Mental illness: a medical condition defined by functional symptoms with as yet no specific pathophysiology that impairs social, academic, and occupational function.

Mental status: a snapshot portrait of one's cognitive and emotional functioning at a particular point in time. It is always included as part of a psychiatric examination.

Metabolize: the process of breaking down a drug in the blood.

Mood disorder: a type of mental illness that affects mood primarily and cognition secondarily. Mood disorders predominantly consist of depression and bipolar disorder.

Mood stabilizer: typically refers to medications for the treatment and prevention of mood swings, such as from depression to mania.

Morbidity: the impact a particular disease process or illness has on one's social, academic, or occupational functioning.

Mortality: death secondary to illness or disease.

Motor cortex: portion of the cerebral cortex that is directly related to voluntary movement. Also known as the motor strip, its anatomy correlates accurately with specific bodily movements, such as moving the left upper or lower extremities.

Neuroanatomy: the structural makeup of the nervous system and nervous tissue.

Neurological: referring to all matters of the nervous system that includes brain, brainstem, spinal cord, and peripheral nerves. Problems with specific, identifiable, pathophysiologic processes are generally considered to be neurological as opposed to psychiatric. Problems with elements of both pathophysiological and psychiatric manifestations are considered to be neuropsychiatric.

Neuron: a nerve cell made up of a cell body with extensions called the dendrites and the axon. The dendrites carry messages from the synapse to the cell body, and the axon carries messages to the synapse to communicate with other nerve cells.

Neuronal plasticity: the act of nerve growth and change as a result of learning. Mental exercise alters neuronal growth in the same manner physical exercise alters muscle growth.

Neuropathic pain: pain secondary to an abnormal state, such as degeneration, of nerves.

Neurophysiology: the part of science devoted specifically to the physiology, or function and activities, of the nervous system.

Neurotransmitter: chemical in the brain that is released by nerve cells to send a message to other cells via the cell receptors.

Neurovegetative: that part of the nervous system devoted to vegetative or involuntary processes such as respiration, blood pressure, heart rate, temperature, sleep, appetite, sexual arousal, etc.

Norepinephrine: a neurotransmitter that is involved in the regulation of mood, arousal, and memory.

Numbing: the psychologic process of becoming resistant to external stimuli so that previously pleasurable activities become less desirable.

Off-label: prescribing of a medication for indications other than those outlined by the Food and Drug Administration.

Overgeneralization: the act of taking a specific event, usually psychologically traumatic, and applying one's reactions to that event to an ever increasing array of events that are not really in the same class but are perceived as such.

Partial remission: symptoms of an illness have resolved by 50%. An impairment of functioning continues to be present.

Pavlovian: from the discoverer Ivan Pavlov. Pavlov paired a bell tone with delivery of food to dogs. The salivation in response to food became associated with the bell over time, such that the food was no longer needed to cause salivation in the presence of the bell tone (see classical conditioning).

Personality disorder: maladaptive behavior patterns that persist throughout the life span, which cause functional impairments.

Pharmacological: pertaining to all chemicals that, when ingested, cause a physiological process to occur in the body. Psychopharmacologic refers to those physiologic processes that have direct psychological effects.

Physiological: pertaining to functions and activities of the living matter, such as organs, tissues, or cells.

Placebo: an inert substance that when ingested causes absolutely no physiological process to occur but may have psychological effects.

Platelet inhibition: referring to the inhibition of platelet activity, such as clotting. Some medications can cause interference in the platelet activity.

Postpartum: referring to events occurring within a specified time after giving birth. Usually within the first 4 weeks.

Pressured speech: characterized by the need to keep speaking; it is difficult to interrupt someone with this type of speech. This is commonly seen in manic or hypomanic mood states.

Prevalence: ratio of the frequency of cases in the population in a given time period of a particular event to the number of persons in the population at risk for the event.

Projected: the attribution of one's own unconscious thoughts and feelings to others.

Pseudodementia: literally, "false dementia." Depression in older persons can cause cognitive effects that mimic dementia. However, in pseudodementia, patients are often overly preoccupied with their cognitive loss relative to patients suffering from true dementia who are often oblivious to their cognitive loss.

Psychomotor agitation: hyperactive or restless movement. It can be seen in highly anxious states, manic mood states, or intoxicated states.

Psychomotor retarded: slowed movement, usually as a result of severe clinical depression. When emotion and cognition become depressed enough, motor function can also become depressed, causing the appearance of physical slowing.

Psychosocial: pertaining to environmental circumstances that can impact one's psychological well-being.

Psychotropic: usually referring to pharmacological agents (medications) that, as a result of their physiological effects on the brain, lead to direct psychological effects.

Receptor: a protein on a cell on which specific chemicals from within the body or from the environment bind in order to cause changes in the cell that result in an electrochemical message for a certain action to be taken by that cell.

Recovery: achievement of baseline, premorbid functioning after successful treatment for a mental illness. Recovery is the term used after a time period of 6 months symptom free. Up to that point, the term is referred to as remission.

Recurrence: the return of symptoms of a mental illness after complete recovery, considered to have occurred after a period of 6 months symptom free.

Re-experiencing: the phenomenon of having a previous lived experience vividly recalled and accompanied by the same strong emotions one originally experienced.

Refractory depression: depressive illness that does not respond to a therapeutic intervention. The term is not typically applied unless such a lack of response has occurred to several different interventions.

Relapse: the return of symptoms of a mental illness for which one is currently receiving active treatment. Relapse occurs during response to treatment or during remission of symptoms. If it occurs after 6 months of successful treatment, during what is termed the recovery phase, the term used is recurrence.

Relative risk: a ratio of incidence of a disorder in persons exposed to a risk factor to the incidence of a disorder in persons not exposed to the same risk factor.

Remission: complete cessation of all symptoms associated with a specific mental illness. This occurs within the first 6 months of treatment, after which the term used is recovery.

Resistance: the tendency to avoid treatment interventions, often unconsciously (e.g., missed appointments, arriving late, forgetting medication).

Response: referring to at least a 50% reduction but not complete cessation of all symptoms associated with a specific mental illness, such as depression.

Ruminations: obsessive thinking over an idea or decision.

Schema: representations in the mind of the world that affect percetion of and response to the environment.

Second-generation antipsychotic: see atypical antipsychotic.

Serotonin: a neurotransmitter found in the brain and throughout the body. Serotonin is involved in mood regulation, anxiety, pain perception, appetite, sleep, sexual behavior, and impulsive behavior.

Serotonin syndrome: an extremely rare but life-threatening syndrome associated with the direct physiological effects of serotonin overload on the body. Symptoms include flushing, high fever, tachycardia, and seizures.

Somatic: referring to the body. Somatic therapy refers to all treatments that have direct physiological effects such as medication and ECT. Somatic complaints refer to all physical complaints that refer to the body such as aches and pains.

Somatoform: pertaining to conditions with physical symptoms thought to be due to psychological factors.

Stressors: environmental influences on the body and mind that can have gradual adverse effects.

Synaptic cleft: the junction between two neurons where neurotransmitters are released, resulting in the communication of a message between the two neurons.

Tarasoff: the name of the family who sued the therapist involved in the care of a young man who murdered a family member. As a result of the lawsuit, therapists are now required to protect and warn potential victims from violent acts or threats made by patients under their care.

Tardive dyskinesia: a late-onset involuntary movement disorder, often irreversible, typically of the mouth, tongue, or lips, and less commonly of the limbs and trunk. These movements are a consequence of antipsychotic use, but are less commonly observed with the newer atypical antipsychotics.

Thought stopping: a technique used to suppress repetitive thoughts.

Transference: the unconscious assignment of feelings and attitudes to a therapist from previous important relationships in one's life (parents and siblings). The relationship follows the pattern of its prototype and can be either negative or positive. The transference relationship is a critical event for the progress of a patient in insight oriented or psychodynamic therapy.

Treatment plan: the plan agreed on by patient and clinician that will be implemented to treat a mental illness. It incorporates all modalities (therapy and medication).

Tryptophan: 1 of the 20 amino acids that constitute the building blocks of proteins in the body. Tryptophan is the building block for serotonin.

Unconscious: an underlying motivation for behavior that is not available to the conscious or thoughtful mind, which has developed over the course of life experience.

Visceral: a bodily sensation usually referencing the gut; also a feeling or thought attributed to intuition rather than reason, such as "a gut instinct."

White matter: tracts in the brain that consist of sheaths (called myelin) covering long nerve fibers.

Index

E

F

G

H

I

Q

R

S

T

U

V

W

Y

Z

June 24